Blessed with a Brain Tumor

Realizing it's *all* Gift and Learning to Receive

Will Pye

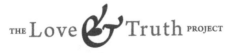

THE Love & Truth PROJECT

www.loveandtruthproject.org

To that which is beyond words, without which
nothing would be, eternal gratitude. May I remember
this presence always.

To Mum, Dad, and Louise -
They say we don't choose our family – if this is
so I am beyond lucky. I love you more than words
can express.

*A human being is part of the whole
called by us the universe, a part limited
in time and space. Humans experience
themselves, their thoughts and feelings
as something separate from the rest,
a kind of optical delusion of their
consciousness. This delusion is a kind
of prison for us, restricting us to our
personal desires and to affection for
a few persons nearest to us. Our task
must be to free ourselves from this
prison by widening our circle of love
and compassion, to embrace all living
creatures and the whole of nature
in its beauty.*

—Albert Einstein

Published by The Love & Truth Project

www.love&truthproject.org

First published in 2014

Printed in the EU by Lightning Source

Typeset by LKSDesigns.co.uk

A CIP catalogue record for this book is available from the
British Library

ISBN 978-0-9929418-0-2

Contents

*Since everything in life is but an
experience, perfect in being what it is,
having nothing to do with good or bad,
acceptance or rejection, one may well
burst out in laughter!*

—Long Chen Pa

It's just a ride.

—Bill Hicks

Introduction

On February 26, 2011, I learned there was a tumor the size of a golf ball in my brain. One might reasonably expect such an event to be laden with doom, gloom, difficulty, and death. Well, clearly no death yet, or else this book brings new meaning to the term "ghostwriting." Perhaps more surprising is the absence of doom, gloom, or difficulty. Indeed, the whole experience unfolded without any stress or suffering. The months following diagnosis were amongst the most wonderful, purposeful, and joy filled of my life. In the years that have followed I have discovered that even the threat of death was not by itself a sufficient motivating force to fully integrate the realizations and insights of those first few months; however, they offered a taste of what is possible and initiated a process through which I am ever more deeply fulfilled, at peace, and in love with life.

At the moment of diagnosis, I experienced deep peace, a knowing all was well. I intuited the diagnosis was somehow a deepening of my journey rather than an interruption, a gift rather than a problem. As I surrendered, I existed mostly on a continuum of joy to bliss, even when, or perhaps because, imminent bodily debilitation and death were possible. Such an experience is not typical. This book will explore how it was possible to respond in this way and how such peace and joy are possible for all of us, in every moment.

The medical opinion was to have surgery immediately, and, given that this was the only item on the medical menu, I chose it. However, days before I was due to have the operation I had an epiphany. I realized that this decision had come from a part of me that wanted to carry on living as I always had, and that I preferred to give the responsibility for resolving the issue to an external authority, albeit in this instance a likeable and highly talented neurosurgeon. In realizing the decision had come from a place of fear and laziness, I decided to take time to allow a wiser perspective to form. In doing so, I sensed there may be another possibility, one that would have greater benefit for myself and society as a whole. To allow time to explore and research this possibility further, I needed to know I was not taking an excessive risk in putting off surgery, and so I insisted on a second MRI scan—it seemed wise to ally intuition with hard data. The second scan showed that the tumor was not growing, and in consultation with the neurosurgical team I chose to postpone surgery.

As immensely intriguing as a "conscious craniotomy" appeared, I intuited more possibility and potential in exploring the creation of a self-induced healing. Following a decade-long quest into the nature of reality, which included the study of mind–body medicine, energy medicine, the phenomenon of "spontaneous remissions," and alternative healing, I was aware that, in principle, by completely transforming the conditions of body and mind which had given rise to the tumor, my body would be able to do what bodies do naturally under optimum conditions, which is heal. My neurosurgeon was supportive of my decision to monitor my brain regularly via MRI scans, respecting that it was my decision to make, whilst being understandably skeptical about the possibility of creating a tumor-free brain without surgery.

I experimented with diet and supplementation, and I made lifestyle changes which minimized stress and maximized joy. I studied scores of books and research papers on the subject, conducted much inner enquiry, met with people who had created their own self-induced healings, studied the modalities they had studied, and had countless healings from alternative health practitioners. There was a degree of success in that the tumor—which we can reasonably presume had been growing in the two years up to diagnosis, was now stable, and regular scans became a formality. My neurosurgeon became more comfortable with my approach—in one report to my GP following our post-scan consultation he stated that *he* had decided I would not have surgery. I was happy to realize that where once he spoke of tumors morphing, he was now willing to put his name to the approach I was taking! In light of the fact that I was not experiencing any symptoms, his view was "We cannot make you any better."

Although I was not able to effect a *reduction* in the tumor mass, I remained confident in my ability to do so. However, as time passed I became complacent and gave less attention to my diet, and I returned to working in the safety and security of my business rather than actively pursuing my life purpose. I allowed old patterns of thought and emotion to resume.

It was clearly time for another wake-up call—I experienced a Grand Mal seizure, and new scans indicated there was a slight shift in the tumor. I remained determined to create a self-induced healing, but a few months later another Grand Mal seizure was followed by a scan which indicated the tumor had grown. The arrival of the occasional headache demonstrated it was time to have that conscious craniotomy I had been so intrigued by.

The operation certainly was quite an experience! I recommend practicing lots of yoga and/or qi gong in advance of the procedure, as being bolted to a hard operating table is uncomfortable after the first hour or two. Despite being immobile, for the majority of the five and a half hour procedure I practiced a conscious breathing meditation and experienced delightful states of consciousness. The surgeon's comment of "That has higher grade written all over it," briefly interrupted my bliss. The pathology results confirmed a stage-three anaplastic astrocytoma. In one moment the probably low-grade brain tumor became cancer, and what I hoped would be the end of this little issue became just the beginning. Half an hour after hearing the news, my father asked me how I felt. I had experienced disappointment; however, I asked again and found peace and joy. On experiencing this at such a time, I was overwhelmed with gratitude—what a blessing!

The mainstream medical menu now offered radio-therapy as a main course, with a possible dessert of chemotherapy. Although there is little sound evidence to support the use of chemotherapy, that I would have radiotherapy was seemingly not in question, although I did ask the neurosurgeon what might happen if I did not.

"You will have problems within months," was the unusually unequivocal response. Thus, having checked in with my intuition I proceeded with radiotherapy whilst also utilizing cannabis oil and experienced no issues other than the loss of hair and an adjusted state of consciousness here or there. The psychological effects of the oil are another story.

As I write this, two months out from radiotherapy and four months from surgery, I am feeling outstand-ingly well. My left hand is now working near perfectly following some minor limitations to spatial awareness post-surgery—on occasion observing me high-fiving my three-year-old nephew it might have been difficult to say who was the more experienced.

Average survival rate from here on in is five to ten years. I will be making far from average choices in terms of diet, daily practice and approach to self and life—there is no room for complacency now—and 20–30+ seems reasonable. At once I surrender such details, trusting life will unfold as it will; my job is simply to enjoy the ride, making the greatest contribution I can whilst remembering what I am beyond and before thought and emotion. This presence, joyful and at peace.

May this book help you gain much of the insight, revelation, joy, and transformative "oomph" of being diagnosed with a life-threatening illness without the considerable inconvenience of actually having one—a sort of virtual-reality wake-up call!

I hope you will also find value as I share the fruits of a decade-long multi-disciplinary, multi-modality, cross-cultural enquiry into the nature of reality and ultimate truth, with a slant towards how such knowledge can help us create the most beautiful future we can imagine.

Where does one look for truth? I tried everywhere. I devoured many thousands of books, blogs, and articles from the realms of philosophy, spirituality, and religion from most eras and traditions. I read self-help books and studied the philosophy and history of science. I explored various fields of scientific research, shamanism, esoteric arts, metaphysics, theology, psychology, ecology, sociology, and history. I read biographies of extraordinary people. I read the novels of the brilliant and the poetry of genius. I explored and experimented with nutrition, exercise, and energy healing. I have been practicing qi gong, yoga and other forms of meditation for over a decade. I tested countless other transformative practices, attending dozens of seminars, conferences, workshops, and trainings. I experienced shamanic practices and plant medicines around the world. I worked with psychotherapists and counsellors, and interviewed quantum physicists, spiritual masters, philosophers, and futurists. I took many long walks in nature.

The quest has been fruitful in many ways. I have healed in myself what psychology would refer to as "depression," and freed myself of various "addictions." In creating my own freedom and well-being, I have found it necessary to look beyond the language, definitions, and assumptions that are commonly used to navigate and explore life. A central message of this book is that how we define events is itself a *creative* process. Science and mysticism (my own and those of every mystic I have ever studied) essentially concur—*there is no objective reality*. All we perceive is but a reflection of the matrix of thoughts and beliefs, images of self, and the world that we have, mostly unconsciously, installed. We are far more powerful than is generally understood. Life now invites more of us to step into this power, not merely for our own fulfilment, but also to midwife a new period of humanity, to birth opportunity from the clutches of the crises we face. As more of us take complete responsibility for our personal experience and the effects of our thinking and feeling, as well as our doing, upon the whole, we will move closer to living in the kind of world our hearts know is possible. We need a new way of thinking to solve some old problems. This book is a modest contribution to our efforts.

How this Book Works

In **Part One: The Seven Gifts**, we will begin with an account of my diagnosis—the events surrounding it and how I experienced them. Each chapter will end with **Questions for Altering Reality**—prompts designed to loosen and open the mind to expand and absorb an upgraded operating system.

Part Two: The Seven Invitations empowers the creation of well-being, creativity, and happiness. Practical exercises are included to facilitate a transformative process. Complete each exercise, because you are committed to living a life of greater fulfilment, purpose and joy; your intention is important. If your intuition guides you to dive deeper into some than others, follow that prompt. Become aware of the distinction between your intuition, (silent, felt, instant) and the resistance of the "ego mind" (noisy, thought and time based). There is no one-size-fits-all miracle cure or tradition, no seven, ten, or twelve steps to happiness and freedom applicable to every unique human in the exact same way. We discover our own approach best by listening to everyone and following no one. We are extraordinarily lucky to live in a time when we can access such a broad range of knowledge. This book distils the most useful and powerful approaches I have discovered and found to be effective in facilitating transformation whilst working with groups around the world. Some will be useful, some less so. Be your own master and expert.

May this book be a contributor to your journey of growth into an ever more fully realized wholeness and joy. May it be an inspiration and invitation to experience yourself as a powerful creative interconnected being, and to continue deepening into the truth of yourself as a source of love and truth in our world.

There has never been a more opportune time to awaken as the joyful being we have forgotten we truly are, than now.

Some big shit will happen …

—Jun Po Denis Kelly Roshi

Prologue

These are not perhaps the typical sage words of a Zen master, but then Jun Po Denis Kelly Roshi is rather more than a typical Zen master. In August 2011, six months before my diagnosis, I was deeply affected by a talk he gave in Australia. Two months later I flew to the United States to attend a *sesshin* (a Zen meditation retreat) in the aptly named Loveland, Colorado. It was in *dokusan*, the meeting between teacher and student, when he spoke the words which begin this section.

That cold Melbourne night when I first heard him speak had found me in the depths of suffering, an angry story of despair replaying in my head. I had contemplated going to a bar that night, but instead I dragged my miserable self to the talk venue. Minutes after Jun Po entered the room, I experienced a profound shift in consciousness. Where contraction and hopelessness had been, now there was spaciousness, joy, and considerable amusement at the melodrama I had only moments before been directing and starring in.

What Jun Po said in those minutes I do not recall; neither do I imagine the *content* of what he said to be of great importance. It was his presence that was so valuable. I recall that, later in the talk, he spoke of how in such "dharma talks" the traditional idea was that teachers would speak to the Buddha statue at the back of the room to symbolize speaking from their Buddha nature to the Buddha nature of each person present. Such symbolism would have usually struck me as merely that, except on this occasion it offered an especially interesting story ... an explanation for this wonderful shift into a state of mind I was familiar with, yet had hitherto seemed so distant from.

Having been passionate about creating positive change in the world for many years, I was deeply moved by the possibility of being able to shift another's state and to lessen their suffering, simply by being present. I decided there and then I wanted whatever Jun Po had. I wanted to be able to bring it online ... to be that spacious transformative presence, consciously and volitionally. I had long wanted to be a source of love and truth in this world, and in offering such presence I sensed how I might be of most benefit. I felt I better understood Gandhi's maxim—"*Be* the change you want to see in the world." I see now how this marked a turning point as I began to shift my focus from working to change the external world to transforming the very consciousness from which the (apparently) external world arises. Starting with my own.

In dokusan, Jun Po continued, "... and you want to be prepared. A sustained meditation practice means we can be useful when such dramas unfold, remaining calm, offering compassion and perspective."

Jun Po was "preaching" to the already converted. I

had practiced meditation (with eyes shut) for several years and was grateful for the huge shifts in my well-being and the insight it had facilitated. In the months leading up to the retreat, I had adopted the eyes-open Zazen practice Jun Po recommends, sitting for an hour or more each day. The eyes-open approach is at once deeply symbolic and very practical. It emphasizes an awake and compassionate engagement with life, here and now, as it is. In addition it is thought to lessen the likelihood of drifting off into pleasing but potentially dissociative subtle states of mind, which are perhaps more likely to occur with eyes closed. This aligns with my own beliefs—what use is "spiritual awakening" if it does not translate into being more useful, more loving, more authentic in each moment of life? Any fool can *taste* and point to enlightenment, but living it—being awake and compassionate, spontaneously alive in each moment, fully embodied and integrated—is true wisdom.

As Jun Po spoke, I found myself agreeing with him. He had been diagnosed with and overcome stage-four throat cancer just a few years earlier. He had experienced so much of life's capacity to throw up vicissitudes of considerable inconvenience that his cancer survival was not sufficiently noteworthy to make it in to his wonderful biography, *A Heart Blown Open.* I imagined the possible dramas he spoke of would be decades away. I would most likely have grey hair by the time a loved one died or I experienced some kind of serious illness myself. Plenty of time to prepare, no urgency ...

Big Shit

The next day, I received a text message from the friend of a close friend back in Australia, requesting that I call at the earliest opportunity. As I waited for it to be a reasonable hour, I wondered what would be the nature of the bad news. I could not conceive of anything positive that would prompt this woman I hardly knew to message me. Why was my friend not messaging me herself?

Eventually, I got through, and I can clearly recall the visceral reaction I felt upon hearing the news that my thirty-four-year-old friend had experienced a stroke whilst driving to work. She had been rushed to hospital, and, following seven hours of emergency brain surgery, doctors now expected—where just hours earlier it had been more a case of hope—that she would live. There were doubts as to what level of brain function and life quality she would experience. As she would explain to me a few months after the surgery, she had been surprised to discover the big black gap on her MRI scan indicating the portion of her brain that had been surgically removed in the life-saving operation. She then surprised doctors, if not those who knew her, by making a rapid and full recovery, relatively soon walking and talking with as much grace and eloquence as before, and returning to work within six months.

It was agreed that I would come back to Australia as planned, when the retreat finished in a couple of days, as doctors were not allowing visitors in those early days. I was able to continue practicing being fully present. This practice would prove to come in very handy in the following months! First, I found myself emotionally collapsing at the next "sharing" in the retreat—so very un-Zen—as I recounted the news I had received and revealed the distress, fear, and sadness pulsing through my being. I was deeply grateful when the group, in our circle, took a moment to envision my friend in good health receiving our love and compassion. How prescient had Jun Po's words been, I thought. Within months this became truer still.

More Prescient Wisdom

It was four months after my friend's stroke, and I had been back in Canberra for some time, enjoying the tail end of a beautiful Australian summer. My friend was doing wonderfully well, all things considered, and I regularly visited her on her family's farm. Hopefully being useful, I helped her to relearn basic tasks and generally offered compassionate support towards her empowered and positive approach to recovery. As a yoga teacher and student of physiology she knew a thing or two about the body. She also brought the same positive attitude and energy to her recovery as she had previously brought to a successful work life.

My friend and I had both long been interested in health, well-being, and the power of the mind. My par-

23

ticular obsession was the nature of reality itself, and I saw my studies as leading towards a deeper understanding and eventual realization of what this life was all about. For a long time I had been collecting quotes of wisdom and inspiration ... words that offered insight and captured essence, typically from great scientists, spiritual teachers, authors, and philosophers. I had a scrapbook full to the brim with such words, and in more recent times had created computer files with quotes on love, truth, transformation, and the like. It was a common experience for me to read a quote and be moved by it. However, on Wednesday, February 23, 2011, I experienced a different category of reaction altogether.

That day I read a quote that did not appear to express anything new yet it induced an exceptional reaction. I experienced a stirring in the middle of my chest. "Yes! That's it! That nails it!" I thought. The profound eloquence of the words—which I have since discovered to be a Buddhist saying attributed to multiple individuals—reverberated through my being: "Death is certain, its timing uncertain; so, what is important now?"

Such a powerful pointer! I felt a deep resonance with getting on with living my most joyous and authentic life. I had completed much successful transformative work and created significant shifts in how I showed up in the world. It was clear, too, that the distance between values and choices, actions and intentions, vision and reality, in each case, was less than I had once experienced. Yet I still felt keenly that I was bringing forth but a fraction of what was possible. I felt challenged and inspired to look more closely at how my life itself answered the question. Beyond my many words, what did my life itself stand for? I had for a long time asserted that I sought to be a source of love and truth in the world, but to what extent was this expressed in my daily life? I shudder as I consider the chasm that existed between saying and doing, talking and walking.

Inspired to a deeper level of pondering, I wrote the quote down in my journal, and it was the only entry for that day. I added no commentary or summary—unusual for one prone to verbosity!—feeling it stood well alone as words of true wisdom. In addition, I would write nothing in the journal for the next five days, the only occasion in that journal in which more than a day or two had passed without an entry filling pages. As is so often my experience, I was excited and inspired by the prospect of more transformation and growth, and guided by the pertinence of the questions. I would soon discover just how pertinent.

More Big Shit?

A few days after reading the quote, on February 26, 2011, I was working out in the gym at an apartment complex in Canberra. Having completed a weights session, I was enjoying a run on the treadmill—so much so, that, when my planned twenty minutes elapsed, I decided to increase the pace and push on. Unlike the day two weeks before when I had experienced what I now know to be a partial seizure—or mere "muscle spasm" as my doctor had unhelpfully described it—I was feeling energized. A few minutes into my extra push, I felt a tingling in my left hand and a mildly altered state of consciousness reminiscent of that which I had felt prior to the partial seizure. In a flash it became very clear that something was fundamentally not as it should be. I began to slow down the machine. It was taking too long, so I jumped off. I was initially able to control the movement, and then gravity took over, and my unconscious body fell to the ground. My next conscious awareness was of sitting cross-legged on the gym floor with two fellow gym goers joining me in a slightly peculiar gathering. They offered me water and explained that I had experienced a seizure—a full-body, convulsive seizure, no less. After they had filled me in on what had happened, I began to get up with the intention of thanking them and returning to my apartment. They gently explained I should probably stay sitting down as an ambulance was on the way. *Oh!*

I was soon on my way to hospital.

On arrival, I sat in a wheelchair for a while feeling quite peculiar. After a short wait, I was given a CAT scan. The kind, female doctor came in not long after to share the results. Her face told me it was not good news.

"There is a lump in your brain," I think she said.

"Oh!" I may have replied.

I have forgotten the details of the dialogue, yet I can recall the doctor's troubled face quite clearly. She explained that I would have an MRI to obtain a clearer picture of what was happening, and I would need to attend another hospital to facilitate this. She was sorry, she said, and left. I was touched by her concern. And immensely intrigued by this turn of events. There was peace, equipoise, and a complete absence of vexation. This may or may not have been related to the effects of the morphine!

At a little before midnight, I was transferred to another Canberra hospital, twenty minutes away, where I stayed overnight. The next day I received an MRI scan; a meeting with a friendly neurosurgeon ensued. He handled the situation in a most casual way, remarking almost flippantly, "We can take it out Friday if you want!" I both enjoyed and appreciated his attitude as it was matter of fact rather than making it into a problem. He also avoided the projection of his fear or death anxiety which can occur when healthy people speak to people whom they know have a life-threatening condition. That was on a Sunday.

The diagnosis, that the lump was probably an "astro-cytoma" or low-grade glioma, indicated a better sort of brain tumor to have; however, the doctors could not be sure. I was advised that a biopsy is generally considered to be too invasive in such circumstances. The tumor was largely a cyst, about five by five by six centimeters. My consultant explained that surgery was the only option, and that it would be a relatively simple operation, lasting about four or five hours. The risk of death was small, apparently, although there was a good chance I might experience some retardation in motor function, which may or may not last. I suggested this last point would be no issue, as I would simply be able to train back anything that was lost. The neurosurgeon responded, "Well, unfortunately, at thirty-one, you are old in neuroplastic terms."

Having studied mind–body interaction, neuroscience, and consciousness for several years, I was aware this point of view was no longer as true as it was once thought. Recent research, which just so happened to have been part of my reading in the previous months, strongly suggested that the extent of neuroplasticity has been underestimated, and that it occurs even into the ninth decade of life in some instances. Our brains are being discovered to be far more malleable and capable of adjusting to environmental stimuli than we had concluded.

I suggested this to the neurosurgeon and let slide his wishy-washy "I'm a sceptic" response, as if we were talking about UFO sightings rather than peer-reviewed scientific papers. I figured it was best to keep on the very good side of a man who may soon hold a scalpel to my brain.

It all seemed to be fairly good news. Being an optimist by both nature and training, I assumed that it was one of the less-threatening types of tumors, and that it would not morph into anything more alarming.

A funny coincidence occurred during the consultation with the neurosurgeon. Following her stroke and surgery, my friend had been placed on an anti-seizure medication, phenytoin, which had caused all manner of unpleasant side-effects. The name had thus been seared into my mind, it being so often referred to in our conversations as the source of all evils. The neurosurgeon explained that they had some anti-seizure medication for me to take.

"It's phenytoin, right?" I inquired.

"Yes, it is," he confirmed, appearing somewhat surprised as he looked up to see my smiling countenance. I was appreciating the irony of a good cosmic joke. I assumed I would experience no side-effects, which proved to be the case—it pays to learn to consciously utilize the placebo effect.

I was discharged the next morning, pills and prescription in hand, with a date for a consultation with the neurosurgeon in a couple of weeks. I had explained to the surgeon that I wanted time to ponder—I would say ponder my options, yet at this stage I did not believe I had any—and develop my understanding of exactly what was happening.

I got home in a surreal haze, stunned by the extraordinary depth of the news. I wondered what to do. I felt no panic or alarm, just immense curiosity. I mean, a brain tumor ... how truly fascinating! I decided to write in my journal.

Opening the pages my eyes fell on the previous entry: *Death is certain, its timing uncertain; so, what is important now?*

In case I might not have worked out the message of the tumor without it, the quote clearly pointed to the diagnosis being my wake-up call, inviting greater urgency to make my life a satisfying answer to the question.

I was overcome with an overwhelming and profound gratitude that such a whisper from the unseen would grace this moment, somehow offering reassurance. I knew that it was all okay, death included, and I had the *experience* of seeing that there is only ever perfection unfolding. I fell to my knees and cried with joy and sadness as a humbling awe and wonder overwhelmed me. And, somehow, from the depths of my being, I knew with certainty what I had already felt—there was nothing wrong. No problem. Just perfection continuing to unfold.

This was the beginning of by far the most interesting event in an already very interesting life. It was the dramatic commencement of a cavalcade of joy, love, and the discovery of why I am really here, what I really am, and what life truly is. Miraculously, this unfolding has been largely free of any stress or suffering and full of gift after gift, which we will now explore.

Our greatest freedom is the freedom to choose our attitude.

—Victor E. Frankl

Part One:
The Seven Gifts

In viewing the diagnosis as a gift and opportunity, I was able to encounter gift and opportunity. Part One shares seven of the most valuable gifts and invites you to give yourself some of the same.

Take a moment at the end of each chapter to ask yourself the Questions for Altering Reality.

Love seeketh not itself to please,
Nor for itself hath any care,
But for another gives its ease,
And builds a Heaven in hell's despair

—*William Blake*

Chapter 1:
The Gift of Love

One of the most delightful and notable aspects of the initial stages of being diagnosed with a brain tumor was an increased and deepened experience of loving, being loved, and *being love*. Being given so much love has been a profound gift. Learning how to truly receive it, profounder still.

Receiving Love

As others became aware that my chances of imminent death had increased, they became kinder. They appeared to look at me differently. Grudges or judgments arising from my past self-righteousness or ignorance seemed to evaporate. Our mortality connects us. The diagnosis of a brain tumor is assumed to be a misfortune, and thus I am offered sympathy. People imagine I must be suffering.

I feel enormous gratitude for this love and kindness shown to me by friends and strangers. We tend to underestimate the powerful impact of a smile offered to a passerby or a moment given to expressing love and appreciation to another. Love has been proven to be a powerful preventative and curative. Our collective health requires a more liberal application of this magical medicine.

One of the most powerfully healing forces of love I received after my diagnosis was from my family.

I love my father dearly. He is a wonderful man—kind, loving, generous, and wise. I looked up to him growing up, and I used to get up early every morning so we could eat breakfast together before he went to work. I would try to eat as many Weetabix as him. I loved to use his breakfast bowl when he was away. I always sought his approval, and especially loved to score a goal in soccer or a try in rugby when he was present to watch. More often than not, he was.

Things changed in my teenage years. I did not approve of my father's behavior regarding my parents' divorce. He did not approve of my taking drugs and generally telling all authority figures (and a particular teacher) to "fuck off!" Talking about emotions is not my father's greatest strength, and the intense anger within me often found no expression. However, he knew I had felt hatred towards him for I expressed this. It is a mark of my father's character that, in the face of great disdain and disinterest from my sister and me, he stuck around and endured the forced weekend trips to the cinema and so on, as we gradually softened and forgave. There was healing still to be done, even twenty years after the breakup, when I was diagnosed.

Who in your life would like to hear that you love them? Express it now. Call, don't text. The book's not going anywhere. Go to the next room and give someone a prolonged hug!

Ten years before the diagnosis, at the age of twenty-one, I had left the UK and my family behind, and over the next ten years my father had perhaps called me twice. We spoke with regularity, but I was almost always the one calling. I sought a closer relationship. I am unusually emotionally open for an Englishman, and so the fit of my needs and capacities has often been slightly off-kilter with those of my father.

Following my diagnosis, he called me every day for two months. Words cannot express the depth of this gift. I learned later this did not yet enable me to truly *receive* my father's love. I discovered that to know intellectually you are loved and to witness this loving in such clear action is still not, in itself, sufficient to create the experience of receiving love. Just as we can have an abundant water supply yet remain parched if we do not turn on the tap, so it is that, in order to receive love, we must remove whatever obstructions we have placed over our heart. In healing relationships with primary caregivers, we become better able to receive the ever-present love of life itself. We do not always see this ubiquitous love; we are like fish who can't see the water they swim in. Often we need first to release a feeling of unworthiness that prevents us from fully receiving. This came later for me and is an ongoing awareness. At the time of diagnosis, the celebration of a father and son's love and its deepening expression was gift enough.

My relationships with my mother and sister also became more openly loving. The love of those around me, and the shifts in many relationships, were wonderful gifts. As we heal ourselves, our families heal, as our families heal our communities heal, and so on. Wannabe world-changers beware—the work must begin with ourselves.

A Special Experience of Receiving

A few weeks after the diagnosis, whilst I was again on meditation retreat with Jun Po, an experience arose that was so delightful it fills me with love and gratitude even now.

It was the closing session of the last day of the retreat, and we each in turn shared insight and reflections. I expressed thoughts on the fragility of life. I was the last to share, and I recall perceiving that Jun Po, when he spoke next, gave my contribution less acknowledgment than I would have liked. I had a sense of not having been heard as Jun Po offered a few words to the group. Perhaps this was a tendency in my psyche to be overly sensitive ... to not receive the love of any father figure. As my own father had once wisely advised, "Perception and reality rarely coincide."

As Jun Po came to the end of his words, he stood up, went into the middle of the room, and asked me to join him. He hugged me and invited others to come join the hug. There was a sweet surreality as thirty or so people joined in one group embrace. Jun Po spoke with an authoritative and deeply loving tone. "Will," he said, "I see you healthy. I see you healed. I see you awake and serving others through your being." He then began a yogic chant, which others joined in with, and at one point a soft female voice soloed a most delightful mantra. The group swayed with a gentle motion, and I moved with them, opening up to this wondrous outpouring of love from a group of mostly strangers. I extend my deepest gratitude to Jun Po and each person on the retreat for giving me such an opportunity to practice receiving.

Giving Love

Just as the more obvious nature of my mortality caused others to be kinder as they became aware that any interaction might be our last, I found myself feeling kinder and more deeply loving. Wouldn't you? What a phenomenal pondering! I invite you to play with it as an experiment right now: Think back to a conversation you had recently. Pick any one. Now, imagine how differently you would have conducted the conversation if you had known this was to be the last time you would ever physically connect with this person. To really ramp up the stakes, consider what effect it would have if you had known this could be the last conversation you ever had with any other human being whilst in this form. Would you listen more deeply? Would you give that person more time? Would you smile more? Would you be a little kinder, and more aware of the other person's feelings?

Now, remember, the possibility of imminent death is true for us all. We have always known this, of course. The Greek writer Euripides wrote in the fifth century BCE, "No one can confidently say that he will be living tomorrow." It's hardly a secret, yet do we live from this truth? It is as if we imagine we will get a card in the mail forewarning us of our upcoming expiration. It is not so. May we live our grandest life, share our gifts, and express our love—*now!*

Let us be reminded that this life is but a fleeting gift. Let us fully unwrap and enjoy this present.

Reminders are all around us. I was chatting with a friend about a meditation retreat I had attended, and I described how an experienced attendee had facili-tated a process by which I experienced an opening of the energetic heart center, which left a physical ache around my chest for days to come. My friend and I pro-ceeded to talk about death in great detail. The next morning I discovered that, at about the same time we were having the conversation, the gentleman who had facilitated the process, Zenrin Jeff Goodman, had died of a brain aneurism. He went to sleep and never woke up. Immediately after I wrote this chapter, LinkedIn asked me if I wanted to connect with him! We are interconnected through countless invisible threads.

We do not need the World Wide Web to connect. We are the Universe Wide Web. Big Love, Jeff.

We can never know when death will come. We rush around, trying to get somewhere other than here and now as if there were anything else. We need not be enslaved by our thoughts, forever missing the wonderfully liberating possibility that this could be the last moment we experience on this planet. Because I have been diagnosed with a potentially life-threatening illness, I find it's not so easy to forget that this moment is precious (yet not impossible). This life is an oh-so-brief flash of the eternal light. These words are a powerful reminder for us all: *Death is certain, its timing uncertain; so, what is important now?*

"Love" is always an appropriate answer! And it is always more important than what we spend most of our time giving our attention to. May we let go of imagined futures and regretted pasts for a moment and appreciate *this* glorious being. Let yourself love being alive.

A great question to ask upon waking is: "Is there someone I would like to share my love with today?" We each have the power to change the world every day by first opening our hearts and then replacing our fear-covering cynicism with naked vulnerability. This is, I suggest for my brothers reading this book, the true measure of a man. As any of the wiser sex may attest, masculinity is not measured only by musculature or the latest car, very nice as these things are! Female and male alike are called to face the world with hearts wide open, available to flow within the eternal dance of love.

Will you remember to give a smile to a stranger whilst out and about tomorrow? Such acts create unseen reverberations throughout the planet, creating joy for ourselves and others.

Anyone who has enquired into life with a little breadth of vision has concluded that humanity is truly one family and community. This is only seen as idealism from a bitterly cynical mind: one too wounded, too fear bound, to see clearly. In our love, our fear, our bodily decay and death, our desire for meaning and connection, we find a shared experience that at once transcends and prompts a celebration of all differences. Our very real oneness is experienced.

Perhaps join me in my daily practice to see and think of everything only with unconditional love. Of course, failure is inevitable, yet the endeavor generates many magic moments.

Choosing Love

Love all that has been created, both the whole and every grain of sand. Love every leaf and every ray of light. Love the beasts and the birds, love the plants, love every separate fragment. If you love each separate fragment, you will understand the mystery of the whole resting in God.
—*Fyodor Dostoevsky*

I have long been fascinated by how we can suffer less pain, experience more joy, and be more loving. I learned that all I need to change is how I am choosing to view the circumstance or person.

I used to become angry when motorists drove in a way that did not meet my expectations, but I discovered that swearing and raging did nothing but generate stress in myself, whilst influencing other drivers to give the same back. So I vowed to change such unhelpful reactions by revising the assumptions, beliefs, and emotional blockages that influenced my unconscious choices. Such a process is simple, if not easy. And once you have made the change, life becomes more fun.

Similarly, I generally no longer suffer or cause suffering when responding to incompetency, either my own or that of others. I have learned to practice equanimity when life does not go the way I would have liked. I am even getting better at "being love" when, for example, a customer service agent at my bank disregards logic or care in our communication. Life abounds with opportunities to practice and grow! And so it was when I was diagnosed with a brain tumor. I saw it as an extraordinary opportunity.

Resisting or denying the undesirable, whether a late train, a coffee that is too hot to drink, the mass of institutionalized greed and hatred, a brain tumor, or indeed our own resistance to the undesirable, only increases discomfort and unpleasantness, and delays the moment we become able to offer an intelligent response.

Denial and anger may be typical stages in reacting to loss or shocking news, with acceptance coming later, after much suffering. However, experience tells us acceptance can, with practice, be an instantaneous response.

Being Love

As you dissolve into love, your ego fades. You're not thinking about loving; you're just being love, radiating like the sun.
—Ram Dass

It is one thing to be loving. It is another order of reality altogether to *be love*. I'm not referring to a nice feeling or weak sentimentality or "romantic love"—a love that is present until something is done that one does not like and is then withdrawn. The love I speak of is entirely independent of circumstances. It is unconditional, for love has no conditions. We might call it "divine love" to give a sense of its proportion, its vast luminosity. It is much more than any one person could take credit for, yet we each have the capacity to embody it. The more established we become in its ever-presence, the more a separate individual constantly driven by what they want or does not want dissolves, and more authentic desires emerge.

This love appears to be a fundamental quality, beyond the normal range of experience. It is hyper real.

This love can be volitionally accessed and allowed to flow through us. There is a stance in life that allows this flow. This stance is loving what *is*. It's very, very simple. Whatever shows up, love it: Traffic light goes red? Love it. Partner does that really annoying thing? Love it. Stub your toe? Love it. Fail to love? Love it. Finding yourself after years of personal transformation coming up against that same old pain or discomfort? Definitely love it.

We can build up to big challenges, such as noticing we are forty-five minutes into a phone call, and through to the fourth department, when all we want is basic information from the bank. Sensing judgment and tension arise? *Love it!* When we experience that horrible, dark, and despairing feeling coming into awareness, try loving it! Diagnosed with a brain tumor? Love it! With such practice, when death comes we can love this too, and the moment of our passing becomes a holy one, minimizing the suffering of those around us.

Three words often follow this challenging notion of extending our love to all that is: "But what about ...?" Typically the question will go on to involve extreme examples such as rape or child abuse or the Holocaust, and to imply that this approach of loving what *is* might involve something other than compassion or that it is a matter of approving of troubling aspects of reality. I have not experienced the challenge of finding forgiveness in response to such cases, yet have encountered remarkable individuals who have. Viktor Frankl was an Austrian neurologist and psychiatrist, and a Holocaust survivor. His brilliant book, *Man's Search for Meaning*, offers an example of how a human can experience the most pronounced and prolonged trauma and yet emerge with compassion not dimmed, but heightened, and with faith and purpose not diminished but defined. His book is guaranteed to inspire; it's a real self-pity buster! I have read of many who in finding forgiveness for their rapist found their own peace. On a documentary a man spoke of how the abuse he suffered as a child contributed to him being the extremely compassionate man he was today. Of course we each respond within our capacities in any given situation. There is no "should" here.

As the gradual development from loving a stubbed toe to loving a brain tumor might suggest, could it be possible to experience *any* difficulty and lessen our pain by loving it?

Love is a complete "'Yes!"—total receptivity and openness. It is an allowing in of every moment, a response to all phenomena, painful or pleasurable, desired or not desired.

Why would you want to take such a stance? Because it deposes suffering and ushers in joy's reign. We discover a curious paradox. When we stop wishing life to be other than it is, our desires are fulfilled. We experience a peace truly beyond understanding.

Whether we call it love or surrender or acceptance, at its heart it is a shift from saying *no* to what is, to saying *yes* to what is. This allows us to experience delight, wonder, and awe as we notice the extraordinariness of every human being. Even being diagnosed with a brain tumor becomes a wonderful experience. This book ultimately seeks to help you to allow more love into your experience and to share that love with those around you. We will explore keys to accessing all this good stuff in chapters to come, beginning with The Gift of Surrender.

Questions for Altering Reality

- *Do you allow yourself to receive the love around you?*
- *Who might you speak to now, and express your love and appreciation for?*
- *Will you first allow a moment to breathe in love for yourself?*

The bad news is you're falling through the air with nothing to hang on to, no parachute. The good news is there is no ground.

—Chogyam Trungpa Rinpoche

When I argue with reality, I lose— but only 100% of the time.

—Byron Katie

Chapter 2:
The Gift of Surrender

Looking back at the experience of my diagnosis, over three years ago, I reflect on its essence. What was the key lesson, the most valuable insight? What allowed it to be such great fun?

And I see clearly the grace that allowed for the peace and joy to surround the experience of diagnosis. It is at once a daily lesson, my life's work, and a moment-to-moment invitation. It is the gift of *surrender*.

An Allegory of Surrender

Imagine yourself in an inflatable rubber ring floating along a "lazy river" in a water park. You cling fiercely to your rubber tube, for there is a nagging sense that without it you would surely sink and drown. You are worried about what is coming up. Other people speak fearfully of waterfalls, screaming children, and other unknown dangers leading to death. You don't recall ever having died before, and although you don't really know what it is, you agree with everyone else that it's scary and to be avoided at all costs. You believe that you need to be in control of every movement, painfully gripping the handles of the rubber ring, but you fail to realize that this control is impossible. Driven by this unconscious fear and consequent desire to be in control, you flail around in panic, paddling this way and that, turning onto your back, your front, and your side, experimenting with different ways of flailing. You flounder in this direction and that, swallowing water here and there, straining a muscle and bumping your head. With minimal success you try to stop the experience at certain points where there is a pleasant view, and speed it up during the unpleasant parts. You believe that things should not be like this. You hope there might be escape—maybe you should obtain a different color tube, or maybe a larger one. So you switch tubes and experience a brief respite from the uncomfortable ride, and you often—subtly and then not so subtly—imply to others that your tube is best. Yet you still complain and moan about the air pressure, the water temperature, and the view.

After much suffering—let's say, for the sake of the allegory, a few hundred times around the river—you have explored all options in an attempt to suffer less, but ultimately none has worked. In desperation, you decide to give up fighting and find the most comfortable position. Lying back, you discover the sky is beautiful. The world now sparkles. All that had been obscured by fret and worry, you now see as miraculous. The ordinary has become extraordinary. You notice you can float even without the tube. You feel fearless. You see that the river takes you where you need to go, and you are perfectly safe. The experience of making shapes out of the clouds enthralls you. Laughter erupts as you realize that all you ever needed to do was to adopt a comfortable posture and cease struggling. This change in posture has changed everything.

This is surrender.

This is where a right-minded human ends up recognizing that our limited perspective of life is simply insufficient to justify arguing with the infinite and eternal mystery. With this recognition, we develop a capacity to consciously respond to events, rather than react through our unconscious emotional conditioning. Mysteriously, the very form of our ever-changing surroundings appears to mirror this newly found ease and joy. It seems that, as we let go and accept what *is*, our experiences become more the way we wanted them to be all along!

From this movement into harmony with life itself, we come to see there is only life that includes the experience of a *me*: I am not separate. I appear separate only in thought. You might see that the idea of falling off a waterfall (and consequently the end of the ride) is for now *just an idea*. It might become obvious there is just one never-ending life, flowing effortlessly, experiencing itself as individuated, as you and me, its destiny, experienced through choice, to realize itself once again as whole.

Surrendering to What Is

Who is surrendering to what? If it helps, consider it might be you surrendering to God, Allah, or the universal Spirit; the small self surrendering to the higher self, the ego surrendering to the soul. Or perhaps we could simply say surrender to what *is*, in its entirety. If talk of God and higher selves troubles you, then let us simply surrender to life. Presumably neither life, God, nor the higher self is too concerned with terminology. Words are important only so far as they help or hinder surrender. How about simply surrender fear for love?

The individual is, as mystics have forever taught, as psychology and neuroscience confirm, and as experience verifies, more than the thinking mind, more than the "me." The exact numbers vary depending on who you ask, but our conscious mind is said to be processing approximately eleven bits of data a second whilst the subconscious mind processes 40,000 bits. In more mystical terms, our personality or ego is clearly finite. It changes and ultimately disappears—in deep sleep, in deep meditation, and in death (allegedly)—whilst what we are, more truly, is infinite. We are infinite being itself. We can verify this hypothesis if we are willing to apply the scientific method within personal experiments using any one of the many transformational paths and processes available to us today. Truth can only be experienced.

The word *surrender* is common in both general usage and particularly within spiritual circles, but the meaning is often misunderstood, and the profound value of assuming such an inner posture is lost. Let's clarify what it is to surrender to life and what it is not. I will first describe how it relates to my being diagnosed with a brain tumor, a case study with specific thoughts and perspectives.

I have heard it said that people respond in stages when they hear they have a life-threatening condition. These stages are similar to the stages people experience at a loved one's passing, which were defined by psychiatrist Elisabeth Kübler-Ross, in 1969, as denial, anger, bargaining, depression, and then finally acceptance.

I have yet to lose a loved one, thankfully, so I am far from expert in this matter. However, I did discover, as I initially interpreted my diagnosis, that I was going to die far sooner than I had thought, so I might assume that I would experience Kübler-Ross's five stages. Somehow, however, I bypassed stages one to four. There was no attempt to wriggle out of the implications or to hope or imagine a mistake had been made. There was no anger. No bitterness. No wishing it were not so. I had thoroughly tested all these approaches to life, and had found them all wanting.

Instead, I immediately accepted that I had a brain tumor, and I recognized all the possibilities this entailed. I embraced the prospect of dying within a few months or years. I accepted my death now. I briefly accepted the possibility of some process of physical and mental degeneration. Beyond this acceptance now, I do not give creative energy to imagining or fearing such an outcome. Death, on the other hand, is rather different.

Whilst possible diminishment of motor function and cognition are specific to the diagnosis of my brain tumor and might or might not occur, death is specific to life and definitely will occur. It is as true for me as it is for you. It is indeed the great leveler. We are, by this measure, living in a world of complete equality. We all might die in days rather than decades. I have been lucky enough to receive frequent reminders via the odd seizure, cranial sensation, and trip to the neurosurgeon. My attention is often on the many aspects of being diagnosed and exploring healing.

I have described the moment of arriving home and reading the quote, *Death is certain, its timing uncertain; so what is important now?* and falling to my knees in the embodiment of surrender. I responded with a big "Yes!" rather than "'Noooo!" It is this acceptance—surrendering to what is—that allowed the arising of joyful peace. When there is nothing we are unwilling to experience, we are beyond fear. We become free from circumstance having any power over us beyond that which we choose to give it, consciously or otherwise. We see clearly that we suffer in the resistance ... in the wishing something was not or will not be. It is in responding that our experience is created.

This is a powerful concept. To live it—to embody it moment to moment—is freedom and joy. Happily, life offers as many opportunities to fall to our knees as we need!

What Surrender is Not

The common usage of the word *surrender* implies giving up or defeat. In the spiritual context, it means the same, yet also much more. In being defeated we experience a most empowered victory. In giving up who we thought we were we gain the vastness of our true nature.

Instantly, by the act of volition, we destroy all suffering. This is epic! It also often arises only after sustained struggle and practice. What, exactly, are we giving up? We are giving up the confusion that the ego—nothing but a desiring and fearing pattern of thoughts—is in control.

We can easily see that the ego is not the master of the Universe. That there are forces beyond us is obvious, bodily mortality being a particularly clear pointer. We might easily grasp that it is a good idea to stop pretending to be only ego. It is a good start to get it theoretically. We can then *experience* this truth. The difference between intellectual understanding and direct experience is akin to the difference between hearing a description of a bungee jump and being tied to a cord, stepping off the platform, and abandoning oneself to freefall. In both "surrender" and "jump" there is a choice point, a critical moment of stepping into the unknown, disregarding the fear and embracing trust instead. The fear becomes elation as we realize the threat was entirely imagined. That choice is the choice to let go, the choice to step into the unknown and discover you are always held. The choice to surrender to life and, by being in harmony with this great flow, be empowered by it.

Of course in the bungee jump scenario the fear is functional. Jumping off high ledges is generally disadvantageous to the body. In surrendering to life itself, however, the fear is *dysfunctional*. That which fears—the ego—has no substantive reality. It is just a movement in thought, helpful for protecting the body and itself, but a hindrance to the experience of what we are. We are neither our bodies nor our minds, but that which sees. In such a realization, we *know*, not by deduction or reasoning but by *gnosis* or insight, that death is nothing to fear, for all that ends is the body, and the mind's chatter. When we are no longer attached to or imagining ourselves to be either of these—the components that die—we see death as considerably less troublesome.

To surrender is a choice. "I" harmonize "my" being with whatever is, rather than follow resistant thoughts. If we were waiting for surrender to be done for us, it would never happen, and we would miss out on the unspeakably delicious experience of reality. Like bungee jumping, such inner acrobatics are not for everyone; however, if you seek truth and the cessation of suffering, surrender you must.

Another reaction to the idea of surrender is to claim that we are endorsing aspects of life that our hearts suggest are intolerable. In fact, we step out of the good-and-bad-judgment game altogether. "There is nothing either good or bad, but thinking makes it so," as William Shakespeare wrote. The process of judging is mere egoic posturing and serves no one but the illusory "me." Plus it is counterproductive, as what we resist persists.

To illustrate this subtle point, imagine we are walking down the street and see an adult ferociously beating a child. Would it be necessary to make a conscious decision as to whether this behavior is "bad" or to consider whether it was legal or not? I would suggest that, for any human of even the most basic capacities, there would simply be a movement to stop the beating. I would suggest, too, though we may or may not talk afterwards about how terrible such things are, at the point of intelligent action arising, there was simply surrender to the scene in front of you. The ego that wants to save the world finds such an idea threatening. However, the world is already saved the more we realize we *are* the world. And solutions naturally arise. And all such confusions of the mind dissolve.

We see that surrender is far from being passive. In allowing what is to be, there is harmony, an inner stance of stillness, alert and active as required. The impact of two of the world's most effective change makers, Martin Luther King and Mahatma Gandhi, shows us that loving what *is* immeasurably enhances our capacity to create change. The energy previously bound up in posturing, controlling, looking good, avoiding looking bad, being right, is freed. The energy, once caught up in maintaining the illusion of the person you thought you were, expresses now through enhanced creativity, joy, and service.

If someone aims a fist at my face and moves it forward at speed, I must first accept that this is so, and *only then* respond intelligently. If I dwell in an inner dialogue that supports the belief that violence is wrong, this guy should know better, and so forth, I will suffer. Surrender does not preclude response; however, it is essential for an intelligent response to arise.

Similarly, if I look at the fact that two billion people on earth live on less than a dollar a day, and I give my energy to ranting about the injustice of this—how wrong it is, that it should not be (the infant's cry of "the world should be how I say it is!")—then I expend energy yet do nothing to alter the issue. Resisting, I give formative energy to that which is. Thus any "war on X" yields the opposite from the desired results. The "war on drugs" and the "war on cancer" are two clear examples of this. A spectacular failure of trillions of dollars and tons of talk as drug use and supply and cancer rates rose dramatically since these initiatives were launched. The failure was in the level of consciousness at which we engaged the issues.

Through acceptance, when we see life is perfect as it is *because* it is, all manner of wonderful opportunities to serve (or to move out of the way of the fist) naturally occur.

There is a subtle yet profound difference between wishing something were not, and envisioning something different. As twentieth-century American futurist Buckminster Fuller said: "To change something, build a new model that makes the existing model obsolete." When our activism is thus informed, when we truly are *being* the change we want to see, we become infinitely more effective.

We don't know how this release of energy resulting from surrender will express, but we can be sure it will be more fun than the resisting and raging.

Surrendering is not just a posture to take with regard to what we see in outer reality. Let's say I observe the judging of my thoughts. Subsequently I bemoan "my" stupidity and smallness. I beat myself up for beating myself up! When I surrender to whatever shows up as it is—and simply observe—I am free to love. Surrendering allows an expansion into being more of what I am.

The quicker we accept *what is* without argument— whatever it is—the quicker the state of mind arises from which change most easily arises. So, rather than surrender being seen as a *threat* to creating positive change, a more beautiful world, a more generous me, a healthier body, surrender is seen as *prerequisite*. American psychologist Carl Rogers summed this up, saying, "The curious paradox is that when I accept myself just as I am, then I can change." Rogers was speaking of psychological growth, however the same applies to how we are creating a more compassionate and functional world.

The Empowering Nature of Surrender

His vast surrender was his only strength.
—Sri Aurobindo

What we have been exploring thus far are mostly mini-surrenders—responses to specific situations that lead to momentary releases and well-being. In contrast, my response to my brain tumor diagnosis was rather more wholesale. I did not merely surrender to the diagnosis and all it entailed, including likely imminent death, but rather I surrendered to life in its entirety, to that which is undoubtedly grander and more intelligent than I am. Indeed I recall thinking something like, *Okay, you got me; you win!* as I fell to my knees in gratitude for the profundity of such an experience and proceeded to consciously give up every single wish, desire, ambition, plan, hope, fear, anxiety, dream, personal development focus, and all that I had ever wanted or not wanted. In this letting go, something miraculous happened. I was no longer obstructed from feeling and being with what is true *now*. And, even more so, what I found to be delightfully true now, beyond ideas, beyond thought, is the most beautifully exquisite joy. Delight. Wonder. Gratitude. Appreciation. Marvel. And all this came not from any accomplishment or practice or experience or circumstance; it came simply from *being itself*.

We will explore this further in Chapter 7: The Gift of Oneness.

The kingdom of heaven is indeed within, and it is here now. We need only give up all notions of "kingdom of heaven experiences" or being happy "in the future." We need only give up the idea of needing anything other than this. Right now. We need only surrender.

If I have come even close to depicting the blissful rapture that followed surrendering to reality as it is, you may be thinking, *Wow I want some of that! Maybe I will try surrendering. Maybe I will give up arguing with 14 billion years of infinite intelligence evolving to this point right now and instead be in harmony with that which is, because then I will get something for myself, and I will feel better.*

This is not surrender! Surrender expects nothing, wants nothing. If we surrender in the hope of feeling good, we are in fact negotiating. Even if it looks like surrender, the results will be different.

So, what to do? Say "Yes"! Say yes to whatever is, and keep saying yes to whatever is, until we are saying yes to life as a whole. Then joy will naturally follow, and, in following where joy wants to lead, we experience all manner of delightful experiences as life around us molds to this new energy. We experience circumstances and situations that we cannot help but say yes to! We wonder how getting more of what we wanted could have involved first giving up all we wanted. More delicious paradox!

Surrender in Action: "I am Yours"

I was brought up in a culture in which God was considered separate from everything, including you or me, and indeed from this world altogether. So long as the divine is separate from me, I can carry on being small. Since these early exposures to monotheistic thought, I have glimpsed the reality in which there clearly exists only the fundamental essence of the Universe, and I experience myself as *this*. Indeed, I realize, via gnosis, that *it* is experiencing itself as *me*. Therefore it becomes perfectly clear that what I am is, one might say, " God godding." This is not a truth which can be arrived at via science, for the subject matter here is infinity—that within which science and all else arises. Neither can this truth be found through the words of others, including those you read in this book. This sharing or any poetry or mystical testimony can, at best, serve as postcards of remembrance of a placeless place. Indeed a place that we never left, though in experience we most likely have forgotten.

In seeking God, Enlightenment, or Truth, we are seeking to remember our very own source, to become intimate once again with a nirvanic emptiness, the heavenly realms that we are. Whether you understand this to be Oneness, God, Consciousness, Gaia, Emptiness, Samadhi, the Self, or your alter ego, Steve, is not as important as public debate would suggest.

It is important to understand that this matter has

nothing to do with *believing* in God or dogma or hypotheses. This is a hyper-rational and empirical enquiry. We are interested here, as grandiose as it might sound, in *God-realization*, rather than mere proselytizing. I hope that, as I share how this often very silly Willy, full of inestimable ignorance and the like, can experience this apparently lofty realization, you will be heartened to ever more fully discover the divinity within you.

Even as the glimpses of ultimate reality broaden into stunningly delusion-shattering rays of truth, and there is only oneness for protracted periods, beliefs and self-images typically still linger or re-emerge. I have found intimate relationships to be a most wonderful means of exposing where shadows or forgetting remains. We learn to welcome these apparent regressions too as we realize that "...*everything* that happens is gently planned by One whose only purpose is your good." (Taken from *A Course in Miracles*, italics author's own.) To return from the depths of being, having looked God in the face and realized you are She—or *it*—might be an extraordinary letdown if we were to resist the experiences of returning. Rather, we might marvel that this infinite and eternal *Being* could experience itself as a separate being in the first place, then awaken to its true nature through the prism of the "I am" sense, and *then resume being a* me *from these previously illumined heights*. From here it is the sense of being me rather than any concept of enlightenment that is most exquisitely wondrous.

How, on earth, did Life do that?

One such experience arose post diagnosis. The recollection sends shivers down my spine.

The vast emptiness which resulted from surrendering to my death had given way to a resumption of the "I am Will Pye" game, in which for moments at a time this ephemeral personality was convinced of its ultimate reality. Observing behaviors and attitudes which, based on experience, were likely to lead away from the experience of love, truth, and God, I found myself crying out in earnest, "I am yours!"

In this posture, I experienced the apparent reality of my separateness and pleaded earnestly to a godlike being, hiding who knows where. I was surrendering *my* will to *thy* will, earnestly wishing that all my petty desires, stubborn habits, selfish tendencies, and profound ignorance would be washed away, and that this God would do with me as it wished. The results would surely be more divine.

A wonderful thing happened: I received a reply.

Just as *I* said to *It*, "I am yours," *It* said to *me*, "I am yours." Simultaneously, in a flash of the infinite, subject and object, self and other, I and it collapsed. There were just a few giddy moments of this glorious being reveling in its own divinity. Yet more gift! An echo of childish conceptions of ultimate reality were gently shattered in one illuminating moment. Life was never the same again, yet changed not one bit. All continued much as before, including the occasional arising of echoes of childish ideas and beliefs. However, now, should I seek to surrender to *That Which Is*, I am reminded I am, most truly and deeply, already one with *That Which I Surrender To*. In the kingdom of Truth, paradox reigns.

Surrender in Action 2: "Jesus, now!"

Another moment of surrender occurred when I was alone in a hotel cabin. I had spent the day in the beautiful New South Wales countryside west of the Blue Mountains and had made myself cozy by turning on heaters, putting on another pair of socks, and rugging up. All was well.

Suddenly, I felt the sensation in my hand and the altered state of consciousness that I was familiar with from the partial and then full-body seizures I had previously experienced. However, this was new territory, for I was not in a public place where a collapsed body might be noticed and aided, but quite alone.

"Oh, shit!" quite nicely sums up my perspective.

I called out, "Help!" and then I called again. The words trailed off as normal consciousness dwindled. I had seemingly lost the capacity to construct words and was falling to the ground. Then it became really interesting.

"Jesus, now!" I said.

What!?

I was calling out to Jesus, not exclaiming, as in "Oh, God!" The tone was not of petition, but demand. I expected a positive response!

The next thing I knew I was waking up the following morning, tucked up in bed with no memory of how I got there, mightily relieved, and somewhat confused.

How might we explain this in someone of no religious beliefs? As echoes of subconscious conditioning perhaps? This does not convince. As a young child, I dutifully attended church services at Easter and Christmas. Indeed, in accordance with the social norms of a good mother or father at such a time and place, I had been christened. The usual God story—heaven and hell—ran quietly in my cultural background. Yet my parents' lack of conviction was clear, and I experienced no encouragement from anyone to believe in anything.

In my teens I had reasoned myself free of the nonsensical blasphemy of most religions I encountered—the usual "only my God is real" or "God is loving yet violently vengeful" doctrines. As I explored spirituality I was repelled by anything Christian as I associated it with judgment, hypocrisy, pedophilia, and guilt. Christianity offered no means or method by which such ignorance could be transcended. I was drawn more to traditions such as Zen Buddhism in which complex metaphysics and issues of faith appear to be avoided and one is simply encouraged to sit down and shut up for a few thousand hours and notice what has always been here.

Furthermore, in the form Christianity took in my young world—that is, the Church of England—Jesus was less prominent than God. Up until the age of thirteen, I had occasionally prayed, when I was really desperate, but I had never prayed to Jesus. I had always, as it were, gone straight to God. And I had prayed to God for only one thing with any persistence—that my parents did not divorce. Upon noting the complete failure of those petitions, I had given up on the game altogether. Whilst it is intriguing that I resorted to *any* relic of my sparse childhood religious education when I found myself in dire trouble, it seems inexplicable that it was Jesus to whom I turned. A merely psychological explanation does not fully satisfy.

My "prayer" having been uttered with such fervor intrigues me further. My tone was strident, even, dare I say it, certain. It was the way one might imagine the tone of someone who had sought divine intervention previously and had success. Confidence of a positive response was high—there was faith. Yet I was not aware I had any faith—and certainly not in Jesus. My enquiry had allowed the certainty only that there was *something*. Something more than we saw or spoke of.

Of course there are a hundred interpretations of the data. My own have deepened on further reflection, yet this book is not the place to delve deeper. For now I share this experience as an intriguing detail of the narrative. I am, of course, deeply grateful for waking up.

Surrendering to Surrendering

It is nice to think that, after one enlightenment experience or dramatic falling to our knees, the job of waking up is complete and we can simply get on with enjoying the bliss and unitive freedom of a life lived *in* and *as* the flow. This generally is not how it pans out; it certainly wasn't for me. The experience of separateness that surrender puts an end to, the experience of ego identification by which I imagine myself to be my thoughts rather than the subjective awareness in which my thoughts arise, are both well ingrained through eons of the evolution of consciousness and conditioned within a Western culture, a culture that is perhaps as hyper-individualized as any culture has ever been. I have heard it said that we are as far from Spirit as it is possible to be. We have journeyed so far into separation we can go no further. The only route now workable is back home into community and unity.

Surrender is one means by which the process of reuniting with what we are is catalyzed. It is easy to see that when we identify with and live from the infinite process of creation (that is, Life Itself), rather than from our finite mind, we access an expanded perspective and understanding.

If I find myself suffering, I know it is time to let go, to surrender. If I find myself believing that whatever may be occurring is a problem, I need only surrender to whatever *is* and to love it. Through my surrender, an infinite spaciousness arises, tinged with a delight in "beingness" itself, and I am able to release any contraction through laughter. It's all very good fun, and the sooner we let go of any identity of being enlightened or any similar idea, we can surrender to this ongoing surrendering that is the key to awakening, and shift the center of gravity from *me* to *we,* from the finite to the infinite, from circumstance-dependent happiness to limitless joy! And then back again, as the spiraling of awakening through apparent time continues.

Lest this seems like a merely personal matter, I would suggest that the future well-being of the human race depends upon such opening. Your awakening to the deeper truth of who you are is the foundation of a new consciousness, a new level of thinking and being, from which our species' not-insignificant problems may be solved. Your personal growth is an impersonal matter. Individual liberation and collective evolution are two faces of one process.

What small stuff can you try saying yes to? In the next chapter we will look to an apparently big deal— death—and the gifts to be found in embracing this too.

Questions for Altering Reality

- *What experience of present pain or challenge might you surrender to?*
- *Might it be easier to align with life rather than oppose it?*
- *Does accepting what is feel good? How does it compare to resisting?*

We are having a hard time living because we are so bent on outwitting death.

—Simone de Beauvoir

To fear death, my friends, is only to think ourselves wise, without being wise; for it is to think that we know what we do not know. For anything that men can tell, death may be the greatest good that can happen to them, but they fear it as if they knew quite well that it was the greatest of evils. And what is this but that shameful ignorance of thinking that we know what we do not know?

—Socrates

To the well organized mind, death is but the next great adventure.

—J.K.Rowling

Chapter 3:
The Gift of Death

According to the old saying, there are only two things to be sure of in life—death and taxes. Yet we spend so much time and energy seeking to avoid both. Clever accounting might help with the latter and yet we remain idiotically determined to succeed with the former. Clever minds even suggest that, in our generation, we will see a cross-fertilization of nanotechnology, artificial intelligence, and epigenetics that will ultimately render death avoidable. Here we see the ego's perennial struggle to maintain itself.

What glorious folly! Death may be a major inconvenience to one's schedule, but it seems also to be rather essential to life. As capital letters and full stops are to this paragraph, death is to life. Perhaps in the eternal unfolding, death serves much the same function as punctuation—to reflect on what has gone before and prepare for what's coming next.

For now, at least, death remains an obligatory part of life. A brain tumor increases one's chances of dying in the short term, yet causes no change to the overall odds.

Generally death is surrounded by much fear. Is such fear necessary or appropriate? Beyond the functional fear which prompts us to steer clear of fast-moving objects and long drops, of what are we fearful?

One might say it is fear of the unknown. And, while some like surprises, others do not. Yet with death, as with surprises, it might be a rather fun experience.

What is Death?

Death is not the opposite of life, but a part of it.
—*Haruki Murakami*

I grew up, as did so many others, with the notion that death was rather like the end of a big lesson for which I had received no schooling. I would end up in either a very nice or a really terrible place dependent on a very complex and slightly mysterious calculating of total murders and masturbations. This, of course, would be weighed against acts of kindness and even what religion or sexual preference I had been born with. Ideas of both heaven and hell as physical realities seemed a little far-fetched. The perpetuation of such a myth is surely sustained only by positing hell as punishment for disbelieving. Fear of loss sells cars and religions alike. Thus religious myth lingers far longer in minds than it might otherwise, as people seek to reason and intuit the nature of reality.

The other main option I considered as a curious

youngster was that death was simply a physical end. If I am merely a physical being, my experience of *me* nothing more than an epiphenomenon of brain activity, then death is the end. I recall this idea of a complete end of me—and thus a total nothingness existing—as being particularly fascinating to my young mind. How consciousness exists at all is a problem within the beliefs of science. How does something come from nothing ... the immaterial arise from the material? This is the "Hard Problem" as Australian philosopher David Chalmers coined it. Well, as a child, I experienced the Hard Problem inverted—how does this something become nothing?

Try to imagine nothing. See if you can conceive of nothing in your mind. I assume that you will discover it is impossible, because anything that can indicate nothing is already something. Even a child's free-roving mind cannot perceive nothingness. Perhaps this is the ultimate koan-like sword with which to cease discursive thought. A koan is a question within Zen without an answer reachable by logic or reason. The answer is found not by thinking it through, but by piercing through thinking to the vast expanse beyond.

I would suggest, as with all problems, that the pursuit of nothingness results from false premises unconsciously informing the perceptual process. In this case the false premise is that we are material beings, and our experience of being conscious is a consequence of the brain. Turn it on its head and see the brain and all else resulting from consciousness, and there is no problem to be found. It is precisely this view that science is slowly moving towards as materialism collapses under its own incompleteness. To look at the research coming from quantum mechanics, neuroscience, epigenetics, and indeed such phenomena as the placebo effect and the various strands of parapsychology, makes materialism sustainable only as a stubborn, not to mention unscientific, belief. Yet this is the lens through which the vast majority of people, even those schooled in reason, regards the world. Part of our evolution necessitates a fuller commitment to reason and an evidence based worldview. The evidence is we are immaterial beings, with the universe more like a mind than a machine. This is something every great scientist from Newton to Bohm to Planck to Einstein intuited.

In my youth, the thought of possible nothingness made death seem far more interesting than disturbing. I would continue to ponder such matters without gaining much clarity, and, like most young people, I lived with death as merely that—an abstraction to be pondered in one's spare time rather than a reality to be too concerned with.

Short answer: I don't know, I am intrigued to find out, yet in no hurry.

Practicing Death

Die before you die.
—*Sufi saying*

Die a little death every day.
—*Buddhist saying*

In my twenties, I flew as often as four or five times a week, and I noticed that encountering the juddering effects of turbulence would elicit a physical fear and discomfort. This intrigued me—was such fear functional? I saw an opportunity for insight, and in response to turbulence I would run different scenarios in my mind in which the plane went down and I faced imminent death. Enquiring whether it was really appropriate to be scared through such thought experiments, I found it was both possible and preferable to be relaxed when turbulence arose. In addition I would ask myself whether had I known such a death were imminent, would I have lived differently? I would typically answer yes, then carry on living much as before, the insight somehow left up in the sky.

This may not sound like everyone's idea of a good time on an airplane; however, I found it a fruitful practice. This ongoing enquiry meant that when faced with the possibility of imminent cessation following the diagnosis, there was no drama. To face death with equanimity is a gift for all involved. Through minimizing stress it is health-supporting. Rather than wasting time and energy wishing the tumor did not exist, or stressing about what might happen, there is an open space into which a more productive way of relating to the circumstance can arise. Consequently, not only was I spared the stress and discomfort of resistance and fear, but also I observed potential gifts, and there was freedom to recognize and receive them in the infinite spaciousness of allowing.

Paradoxically, the relaxation elicited by acceptance is likely to create an improvement in physical health. Psychoneuroimmunology has long proven this, and it is particularly well surmised by the work of American researcher and cardiologist Herbert Benson.

What is Important Now?

How often do we hear of individuals for whom facing the specter of death prompts an improved prioritizing of what is important? It seems that once death is no longer possible to ignore, and the delusional thought that we can "always do it later" is laid to rest, hindrances and obstructions within the mind are lifted. We regard life as it really is—a precious yet fleeting opportunity to express and experience our heart's desire. Perhaps this is the great gift inherent in such circumstances, yet the speed and ease with which we receive it is determined by how rapidly we are able to open to the reality of our mortality. Is that a good reason to make peace with your death at the earliest opportunity?

In my experience, making peace with my own death has led to a number of wonderful developments, the first of which—experiencing myself as that which does not die—is rather fundamental and underpins all the others. Chapter 7: The Gift of Oneness will explore this in more depth. For now, I'd like to focus on a particular gift that arises from accepting that it could be all over in a moment. This is the gift of joy.

When I experience "this moment" as possibly my last, the extraordinary wonder and beauty that is always present becomes crystal clear, and the ordinary phenomena of manifestation and form take on a gloriously wondrous sheen. I realize this inherent delight is in the fabric of life itself—in things as they *really* are, as apart from what we *think* they are. This luminescence is as much visible in a lamppost or fecal matter as in the more obvious examples of a child's smile or a pretty sky. All we need to do is see clearly and perceive directly rather than through the skewing filter of mind activity. The big question is: *How* do we do that?

"Know thyself," said Greek philosopher Socrates way back in the fifth century BCE. As you are infinite, don't expect this task to be completed anytime soon.

A good starting point is to check whether our filters—our beliefs and personal narratives about life—are true and helpful. Do they help us create what we want in terms of experience and response? Having begun our work here, we move beyond the filtering of mental activity—ruminating, speculating, and projecting this and that—to perceive life as it is, clearly and directly. A consequence of so doing is coming to the same realization articulated by countless visionaries, mystics, poets, and inspired scientists—that *this and that* are, more truly, just *this*: that beyond the very helpful separating and distinguishing functions of mind, there is just one whole, and this includes us—we are not apart from it. We experience unity.

A fruitful practice for me has been to shut up and sit down for a while. (Perhaps a few thousand hours. You may be less obdurate than I and require fewer hours.) I have enjoyed doing so within a Zen context. However, one can use whatever works. If you are impatient, brave of heart and relatively sound of mind then Life has been kind enough to create many an entheogen (plant psychotropic) that can offer this vision of unity. In my experience, a meditative practice, along with the use of such catalyzers as psychedelics or transformative breathing, is ideal. I would encourage only a pragmatic approach; whether you are exploring meditation, entheogens, or breathwork (such as Transformational Breath® or Holotropic Breathwork™), do plenty of research and explore with a teacher or experienced practitioner.

In the journey into vastness, a tour guide is helpful at the earlier stages. Your heart is the only guide you need once you realize you have already arrived. If you believe you need a guru, question that thought; look from where it comes. It might come from confusion as to what you are—confusion many a fake guru has exploited. Guru or devotee: in most cases they are simply different forms of the same ego game. Except when they are not—there are apparently genuine gurus of extraordinary powers and depth; however, they are exceptionally rare. More delicious paradox. Assume any teacher is at best half-baked, at worst a charlatan, until proven otherwise.

It is easy to imagine that in such circumstances of realizing one's oneness with everything—and noticing that this everything possesses an inherent delightfulness—joy naturally arises. I have also noticed that the full apparatus of mind activity—thought, fear, worry, and so on—can reassert itself. Nevertheless, it becomes ever easier to drop back into this ever-present direct perception of perfection. I have been especially delighted to discover that it is possible to *choose* joy!

Thus, facing imminent death gifted both the means and enhanced motivation to experience joy *now*. I have made this the new standard for my life experience. Whilst I have generally not been one to dwell on unpleasant situations, I have become ruthless in this regard, politely ending conversations, leaving cinemas, and discarding books with greater ease and haste as soon as it becomes clear they do not contribute to my joy and well-being. Experiencing well-being is the essential foundation from which I can serve other's. We are all of us curators in this world. Why include tedium and triviality in our experience, when more fruitful options are often just a change in perspective away?

I live in a culture that appears confused on this matter. Making such happy life choices is often considered to be selfish. Instead, some say, one should endure unpleasant situations because "this is simply the way life is." Let us be clear that, whilst it is possible to choose an unpleasant life, life itself is quite as happy being a delightful dance of joyful self-discovery and self-expression. Whenever you hear the word *should*, be cautious. I no longer have any need for this word. It has withered away as its gnarly roots of fear, control, and self-righteousness have diminished. "Quit should-ing on yourself!"

What is especially wonderful about engaging with life in such a way is that one naturally and effortlessly becomes a useful source of joy for others. I would encourage anyone wishing to serve others to truly serve themselves first. Just as when you're in a threat-ening situation on an airplane you must put on your own oxygen mask first before you help others, in life we discover our own peace and happiness before we can be of greatest help to anyone else.

Paradoxically, an essential part of being at peace and in well-being is the capacity to feel and experience the full range of emotional content and to bear life's challenges and difficulties with equipoise. There are times when we simply need feel what is to be felt; this capacity to embrace all that arises with an open heart is a life practice. To be unattached to joy or despair, to life or death, is real freedom.

Rather than doing what I *should* do, I now do what I *love* to do. Before diagnosis, I had long worked in the very rewarding and challenging arena of face-to-face fundraising. This allowed me to grow daily and to over-come my limitations whilst helping others do the same and contribute essential funding for many great service organizations so that they could fulfil their missions. However, what I had always really longed to do was to effect change at what I see as a more fundamental and thus causative level of reality: the level of thought, of consciousness. Here ideas, thoughts, and feelings are the formative matrix that leads to individuals, and thus societies, thriving in a healthy world, conscious of our interdependence and shared oneness.

I now coach, write books, lead workshops, speak at events, and make a living doing what I love. Before the diagnosis, I only dreamed of such wonderful possibilities. It's amazing what a sense of urgency can do! Looking back at this most creative and authentic period of my life, I can only feel great gratitude for the gift of death.

An Almighty Inconvenience

So, what is death? If Buddha himself is said to have chosen not to answer such a question, then perhaps I would be wise to do the same. I have my ideas and nice narratives, yet I realize they are but that. With this question, as with all life's big questions, the only really useful answers are those we come to realize ourselves. Ultimately I would encourage anyone investigating the nature of death to include in their research the data surrounding near-death experiences—a section of titles is included in the Further Reading section at the back of this book. If we read with a willingness to let go of preconceptions, we may find new ideas illuminating. As our meditative practice deepens, we might gain further insight. It's remarkable what emerges when we create the space in our minds.

We do know death happens. Let us assume we don't know *what* happens. Why would we fear that which we do not know?

Sure, we might insist on fearing not having what we have. But, clearly, as we have it now, and now is all that exists, that would be unreasonable. Might being grateful for what we have now be more fun? Let us not waste a precious moment!

Just as when we are children we come to know that there is nothing to be feared in darkness itself, we may come to realize that, in the case of death, curiosity is perhaps a more helpful perspective. Like anything, until the actual experience of death arises, death is but an idea. We can choose how to feel about this idea. I reserve the right to scream like a little girl when it happens; however, until then I am merely intrigued, preferring it does not happen for a long time yet.

Being Prepared

In a speech at a Stanford University graduation, the then CEO of Apple, Steve Jobs, suggested that "death is the single best invention of life." Death enhances life by giving reason to get on with doing anything at all. The powerful context of loss and grief ultimately deepens life experience as a whole. And the big questions it creates—whether nothingness can come from something, or, if it can't, what other realms exist—add to life's rich texture.

Jobs shared this philosophy: "I have looked in the mirror every morning and asked myself: 'If today were the last day of my life, would I want to do what I am about to do today?' And whenever the answer has been 'No' for too many days in a row, I know I need to change something."

How about you?

In facing death, we discover it to be a gift. In asking such questions we access the Gift of Guidance.

Only put off until tomorrow what
you are willing to die having left undone.
　—Pablo Picasso

Questions for Altering Reality

- *Death is certain, its timing uncertain; so, what is important now?*
- *What would you change if you knew you were going to die in a week or in six months? What's stopping you from making that change now?*
- *If you are not living in joy, loving what you are doing, and spending time with people you love, how can you change yourself and your life so you are?*

The Realm of God is inside and outside you. (Thomas, 3)

Seek and you will find. (Thomas, 92)

—Jesus

Sin is the idea you are alone and separated off from what is whole.

—A Course in Miracles

*The psyche is the greatest of all cosmic wonders and the "sine qua non" of the world as an object. It is in the highest degree odd that Western man … apparently pays so little regard to this fact. Swamped by the knowledge of external objects, **the subject of all knowledge** has been temporarily eclipsed to the point of non-existence.*

—Carl Jung (Author's emphasis)

Chapter 4:
The Gift of Guidance

This chapter is about how, as a result of asking and being open to how the answers came, all manner of guidance became available and my life's purpose became clear.

In choosing two epigraphs associated with Christianity, I offer the example of how guidance came from *the essence* of a religion that I long ago rejected and the value in keeping an open mind. The epigraphs themselves speak of how life is available to guide our evolution and healing. In realizing that we are not separate from life, we find the reality of there being guidance available easier to grasp. I will offer some of the synchronicities of my own experience as examples of guidance, but first a proviso or two.

A further reference to Jesus here may bring up baggage and confusion. Being associated with a religion can trigger a closing of minds and hearts. However, I suggest that, in discarding Jesus along with the religion which has typically so misinterpreted his teaching and a church which has often so spectacularly failed to exemplify them, we are in danger of throwing out the baby with the bathwater.

In so doing we miss out, for Jesus Christ appears to have been one wonderfully divine dude with a teaching and example of immense value to anyone seeking love and truth, spiritual awakening or a world reborn. The good news is we can access the gifts he shared without having anything, or everything, to do with Christianity.

I respect everyone's right to believe in anything. At once I would assert that, whatever we believe—atheism, agnosticism, the dogma of a particular faith, materialism, the superiority of science over mysticism as a means of understanding the world or of Zen as the most effective transformative path—such belief is unnecessary, and unhelpful if firmly held. To experience Truth or Ultimate Reality, the kingdom of heaven that is within you, involves dropping the mechanism of believing or disbelieving. As with everything in this book, this itself is a hypothesis to be tested in your experience. Let intuition and curiosity be your guides.

Of course, if you believe the possibility of your own enlightenment or salvation to be untrue, as a projection of your own mind, your life will conform and it will remain untrue for you. We have to be open to receive.

The words attributed to Jesus at the beginning of this chapter suggest that heaven is an internal state rather than an external reality and point to an awesome truth—what we experience as "outer" and "inner" are at a fundamental level, one. The experience of you and me that we share in ordinary consciousness is but an appearance overlaying a deeper unitive field of being. Separation, and all its suffering, is a dream. Indeed, everything that we perceive is a dream, and the more we awaken to this, the more lucidly and playfully we can create a more dreamy dream. Perhaps personal and collective crises are part of the mechanism by which the one intelligence facilitates this expansion. We will explore the experience of this ever-present here and now underlying unity, available to you and I, as it was to Jesus, in Chapter 7: The Gift of Oneness. I suggest that this realization is an aspect of an emerging new consciousness, a consciousness we might label "Christ Consciousness." It arises when the confusion and fear of competition and the separate self dies, and is "resurrected" into the joy of unity: *me* realizes it is in fact more *we*. How valuable could such a realization be as we face our collective challenges? How valuable could a deepening of this realization be in our own life?

If we desire this heavenly realm, we need first ask with all our heart and be mysteriously guided, in good time, to the realization that heaven is within. So long as we are in this remembrance, we can do nothing but love our neighbor. Here such conduct no longer need be commanded; rather, it *is who we are, being what it is*. It is our opportunity to bring love into this world par excellence.

Experiencing the kingdom of heaven is a reminder that the immaterial and transcendent heaven is not separate or only accessible after physical death. It is here right now, intertwined with—and is indeed the essence of—earthly life. One of the ways we can observe such a benevolent intelligence is through synchronicity.

Some Guidance from Jung

Synchronicity is when two or more events happen coincidentally in a way that is meaningful to the person experiencing them. The connection cannot be explained causally—there is no apparent way one could have resulted from the other; there is no direct cause and effect. Rather, events are related by *meaning*.

The man who coined the term "synchronicity" was Swiss psychotherapist and psychiatrist Carl Jung. To explain his idea, Jung recounts the story of a patient of his who was having difficulty experiencing a deeper meaning in life. Jung suggests she suffered in this way due to an excessively "rational" bias in her worldview. We might define this as the belief that, if something cannot be seen or measured, it does not exist.

In a psychotherapeutic session with Jung, the patient was recounting a dream featuring a scarab beetle. At that very moment, a beetle—not a scarab, but the closest to it in Europe—alighted on the windowpane in the full view of both the patient and Jung. The patient perceived this as being deeply significant, in particular interpreting it as a message that she needed to open up her mind ... that perhaps there was a deeper meaning to be found in life. It proved to be a breakthrough in her therapy. The topic fascinated Jung and his friend the great Austrian physicist Wolfgang Pauli for years to come.

This example, as I see so often in my personal experience, offers the *transformative* aspect of synchronicities — the fact that there might be unseen, seemingly immaterial activity "causing" the events to arise. It also brings on board all sorts of metaphysical questions and distractions, which trouble the modern mind. Because it is such an ill fit for the materialist dogma of our time, such phenomena (whilst they may be common in personal experience) are not explored as deeply as they otherwise might.

In my experience, however, such phenomena have been a mechanism by which the partial nature of the explanation and exploration of life offered by materialism is exposed. Gradually such experiences eroded my atheistic and cynical view. Eventually they became so startling as to inspire the experiences of wonder, gratitude, and awe that naturally arise when doubt is dissolved by the sheer luminescent obviousness of an immaterial intelligence interweaving the very fabric of our experience. Call it God, Life, Spirit, the Mystery—whatever you like—the revelation is irreducible.

Synchronicity is thus, I suggest, one means by which the unseen manifests in form. It is the means by which the unity that is life intrudes upon the separate "self" experience. As we approach a more unitive consciousness, synchronicities appear with increasing frequency to accelerate our path to joy.

As I share with you some synchronicities that have occurred in my own experience, it will become clearer how the experience of being diagnosed with a brain tumor was so fascinating and enjoyable. Hopefully, this will encourage you to look for similar phenomena in your own experience. Synchronistic events can be of immense practical use when allied with sound reason. They offer clues about how to respond to particular circumstances, in addition to reminding us that we are living an interconnected, beautiful, and meaningful mystery.

Synchronicities I Have Known and Loved

The first synchronicity I experienced came when I was nineteen years old, outside a friend's parents' house in the middle of the city of Cambridge, England, one evening. Following a party weekend, we were adjusting to the reality of the resumption of sobriety and work the next day. My friend proceeded to tell me a funny story involving the father of a mutual friend of ours. This man was known for being very stern and aloof, rarely smiling or even expressing the slightest emotional experience. One night, my friend and our mutual friend believed they had seen an owl in the garden. Upon overhearing this, the stern-faced father had come out into the garden and proceeded to offer an animated and expressive owl impersonation in an attempt to lure the bird. This was very funny to imagine, and we laughed as the images rolled through our minds. Then silence settled. Within a few seconds an owl alighted on the tree a few meters in front of us. We could see it clearly, and it faced us directly. As I recall, this was simply a nice coincidence for my friend. Yet for myself it had great meaning. I could not say why or what.

Whilst the prevalent view within the culture of my upbringing would be that this was "just a coincidence," it was clear to me that this description was insufficient. I simply *knew* it meant something. Prior to this experience, I had been searching for truth; however, it had shown up merely in curiosity as to what was *really* happening within global affairs beyond misspeaking politicians and manufactured consent. Only occasionally would I casually contemplate what death was, whether God existed, and the like. I was looking for truth solely within existing belief systems, generally accepting the implicit assumptions of the materialist worldview. In the years following the owl experience, I began to question these assumptions and came to see their partiality. This introduction to synchronicity was the first stirring of a faint inner call, prompting a deeper exploration of what I am and what it means to be human.

I could *reason* that the event was significant based on the improbability that the only owl appearance in my life would occur within seconds of an owl-centered dialogue. However, this was not how I arrived at the fact that it was meaningful for me. Just as we sometimes *know* or *feel* someone to be a significant person for our future when we first meet him or her, so I *knew* this owl event was significant. Learning to access and trust this inner wisdom—intuition—is a gift that continues to deepen.

Years after the owl incident, I was living in New Zealand and took my partner to one of my favorite spots in nature. We were falling in love, yet I remained hesitant about making any commitment. We were visiting the same location by the Waikato River where the previous day I had been regaled by a fantail bird, dancing all around me with an astonishing intimacy and interest. Whilst such birds are known to be more friendly to humans than most, this occurrence struck me nonetheless. I wondered whether the bird would be there on this day I'd brought my partner, and, if so, would it be as friendly with my partner as it had been with me, an expression perhaps of the doubts I was experiencing about our relationship.

When we arrived, I was delighted to discover not one fantail but two, which then proceeded to dance around us for several minutes, tweeting as they followed us through the undergrowth. The experience was repeated days later. I have not before or since seen two fantails behave in this way. At the time it was *as if* life was responding to my doubts with the most beautiful confirmation that this partnership was indeed part of my unfolding and served my highest good. As fear has fallen away and the old worldview crumbled under its own partiality, I would now remove the "as if."

Some months later we walked through the same area, which had become a special place for us, and I shared the owl story I had experienced when I was nineteen. On finishing the story, I looked up and saw two owls looking down at us from a tree. I took this as confirmation of the deep value of our partnership and as an antidote to the fears and doubts that lingered and prevented a fuller receiving of the available love.

In many traditions, the owl is the symbol for wisdom and transformation, which further imbues these experiences with personal meaning. The owl has to this day continued to be the most common symbol to appear in my synchronistic phenomena.

I have already shared, in Chapter 1, the wonderful synchronicity involving the quote that I had written down four days before diagnosis: "Death is certain, its timing uncertain; so what is important now?" I had written those words into my journal at the top of the page, adding nothing in the days following. I had no way of knowing that these would be the first words I would read after my diagnosis.

Perhaps you can imagine the depth of the synchronicity and ongoing meaning that arose at the time, a meaning proportional to the scale of such a life-altering event as being diagnosed with a brain tumor. What a truly wonderful coinciding. The question, "So, what is important now?" has become a guiding inquiry as the journey has unfolded. It has, on many occasions, brought my mind back to joy and to love, and it serves as a reminder to choose that which best serves rather than repeating old patterns created from fear and greed—maybe when I am aimlessly surfing the Internet or procrastinating over the writing of this book. Or perhaps the question will arise when I'm considering a glass of wine rather than meditating, and I am reminded to choose what I *really* desire and which brings lasting delight—truth, awareness, *being love*. To this day, the inquiry continues: What do I truly desire to do with this life?

In May, 2011, a few months after being diagnosed and the day before my birthday, I walked with my mother to the tennis court in the village I grew up in, passing through the graveyard along the way. A curious sight caught my eye—a headstone for someone who had lost her life on the very day I was born. The stone was standing alone and very prominently positioned in relation to the path. It was impossible not to walk past it. In spite of my mother having walked that path hundreds of times, and having a keen interest in family and village history that would occasionally lead her to peruse gravestones in this small churchyard, it was the first time she or I had become aware of it. This reflected the theme of life and death so alive at this point, reiterating the sense of urgency necessary to create major change. One day, tomorrow will not arrive.

On the next day, the morning of my thirty-second birthday, I was putting down in writing what I really wanted to do in life. I appreciated working in fundraising and being a business owner, yet I knew I was most passionate about the nature of reality and facilitating transformation. I noted two professions which would help me express and serve with these passions in mind: coaching and writing. I then sat down to watch a film, flipping through the fifteen DVDs I had bought recently to determine which was the right one for that day. I was restricted by time, and so searched for those less than one-hundred minutes in length. I found a handful.

One was a DVD I had chosen to watch a few days before, but then decided not to. However, on this day, my birthday, it felt like a good time to watch *Shattered Glass,* a movie about Stephen Glass, a journalist discovered to have made up almost all of his supposedly non-fictional articles for the magazine *New Republic.* One of the dates that came up on the screen during the film was "the day of judgment," when the editors determined how to respond when they discovered his fraud. It was my birthday in 1998. A nice coincidence, I thought.

Following the film's conclusion, I felt intrigued to find out more about Stephen Glass and in so doing came across stories about Jayson Blair, another journalist who was discovered to have been making up stories, this time for *The New York Times*. My meaning meter wagged a little more fully when I discovered that Blair's judgment day, or moment of truth, came when *The New York Times* published a front-page article exposing his deception, on my birthday in 2003. On my birthday, a day on which I was clarifying what is most true for me—writing and coaching—I believe I was presented with two individuals who were exposed as living a lie, events which also occurred on my birthday.

My meaning meter went off the charts when I noted what each was now doing. Glass became a writer; Blair a life coach.

I am now, amongst other things, a writer and a coach!

It has become apparent as my worldview has gradually expanded to allow it—through meditative insight and conclusions as to what the latest scientific data suggest—that I live in a universe where meaning and

guidance is somehow woven into the fabric of form ...
into life itself.

I was in Wellington, New Zealand, enjoying reading
Roderick Main's book, *Revelations of Chance*, which
deals predominantly with the synchronistic material
of two individuals. One was Edward Thornton, whom I
discovered to be, like myself, English, a businessman,
a meditator, and mystic, and for whom the owl was the
central figure in his synchronicities. Main described
Thornton as having a dream about his head being
shaved, which had great spiritual significance for him.
I long ago had a similar dream, which also had great
significance. In addition, Thornton was diagnosed with
a brain tumor and saw it as a great spiritual opportunity. I am happy to say he was cured, via surgery in his
case. May the coinciding continue!

That night I went out enthused and inspired by such
an extraordinary synchronicity. Owls were all around.
Barely had I left the hotel when I noticed a display in
a shop window, one not typical on a city high street:
six distinct and equally kitsch owl figurines. Later that
night my friend and I walked past another shop window and a clock with an owl as its centerpiece caught
my eye. And I was reminded, "So, what is important
now?" The clock is ticking, and each moment we
embody our answer to such a question.

As we look at ourselves we might ask, "Does my
life align with what I say I value and desire?" If it
does, you will likely find yourself happy and in joy. If it
doesn't, you will likely find yourself otherwise. You will

likely agree that it is better to listen and act on our deeper sense now rather than be so stubborn as to require a brain tumor to spur you into action!

Allying a poetic or symbolic reading of life with our reason, and using our feelings as well as our thinking, makes for a more truly intelligent means of navigating life. This integrating of heart and head, spirituality and science, is, I believe, a focal point of the emerging worldview, and a key element of our personal evolution.

More Owl Synchronicities

As my father drove us to his house on the evening I had nearly completed writing this chapter, my mind and talk were awash with synchronicities. Moments after a conversation on this topic with my father, there was a flash of brilliant white swirling alongside the car and then in front of it, flying with us for a couple of seconds. "An owl!" my dad exclaimed as I smiled to myself, feeling connected, guided, and deeply grateful.

A week later I shared this experience with my mum as we were driving along the same road in the opposite direction, and I quoted a line from Japanese writer Haruki Murakami's novel *IQ84*: "The owl is the guardian deity of the woods. He knows all and gives us the wisdom of the night." I related the high prevalence of synchronicities I had experienced, and how I had incorporated them into this book. I spoke of the owl appearing when I had been driving with my father.

A few moments later, an owl flew *out of the woods* in front of the car!

Intriguingly, the next six months were characterized by intense "shadow work." It seemed as if every unpleasant emotion or feeling I had ever not wanted to experience came into my awareness to be owned, loved, and let go. Perhaps, as I interpreted it, the owl's presence was pointing to the necessity of bringing into the light the subconsciously disowned or repressed feelings that would inhibit my physical healing. In such ways are we guided towards greater wholeness and well-being.

Let us truly open our minds to understanding more deeply what is real. Let us allow our own hearts and minds to guide us through our own experiences. Let us explore now that we may ask more clearly, and notice more frequently, the wonderful means by which this benevolent reality guides us towards greater well-being. We need only be willing to ask and listen and discover the Gift of Guidance. If we remain curious, we may notice that the guidance appears to point in a particular direction, and we discover the Gift of Purpose.

Questions for Altering Reality

- *In what ways has life conspired to serve your growth and well-being?*
- *When has something "bad" happened that turned*

out to open the way for a great learning experi-
ence or a change you would now consider "good"?
- *Would it be helpful to notice and appreciate more*
  often how moments of apparent chance can
  serve your growth?

*Purpose is the place where your deep
gladness meets the world's needs.*

—Frederick Buechner

*Don't ask what the world needs. Ask
what makes you come alive and go do
it. For the world needs people who have
come alive.*

—Howard Thurman

The purpose of our lives is to be happy.

—Fourteenth Dalai Lama

*Many persons have a wrong idea of
what constitutes true happiness. It is not
attained through self-gratification but
through fidelity to a worthy purpose*

—Helen Keller

Chapter 5:
The Gift of Purpose

As a teenager, I desired to be rich and to have sex with lots of beautiful women. Yet a deeper purpose was also coming into my conscious awareness. I decided I wanted to be a positive influence on everyone I met. By such a standard, my life would thus be determined successful to the extent that anyone encountering me would leave somehow elevated and better off. This expression eventually evolved into, "being a source of love and truth" in the world. As this purpose crystallized, it was clear this was no mere wish to be nice, kind, and honest; rather, I sought to offer an unconditional love and an embodiment of the deepest truth—to speak, act, and *be* love and truth.

Truth is humble, unattached to any position or opinion, moderate in its desires, and accepting of whatever arises. I had then—and have now—a long way to go. The journey towards these ambitious outcomes has involved experiencing fully arrogance, self-righteousness, greed, hopelessness, and hatred, mostly against myself, but which I would at times project out on to the world.

For ten years prior to my diagnosis I had been

investigating the means and methods by which this ultimate goal might be achieved—how to heal and transmute the negative energies of the mind, how to dissolve the obstructions to my heart and enlighten the darkness obscuring my soul. The diagnosis provided the impetus and provocation to get on with this task with a renewed vigor and fuller commitment. Following the first seizure and then again after the most recent seizure, which led to the MRI that revealed that the tumor had grown—at a point when daily commitment to this endeavor had been flagging—I was guided by that powerful question: "So, what is important now?"

A great gift of the diagnosis has thus been the transformation of my life into a more convincing *living* in answer to this question. This is the gift of purpose—discovering my life's purpose and deciding, once and for all, to prioritize living it.

We are each here for a special function, a particular expression of our gifts and passions. Our weaknesses and frailties are a necessary part of the alchemy of being by which we come to most fully express this purpose.

Mozart was already expressing his at the age of four! For him it appears there was no period of searching or seeking what it was he valued most or what he was here to do; rather, the appearance in his consciousness of complete symphonies of genius made it clear. The tightrope walker Philippe Petit, featured in the beautiful film *Man on Wire*, realized in a dentist's waiting room in 1974 that his reason for being was to create a masterpiece—walking a tightrope between the two towers of the World Trade Center. Gandhi discovered his real reason for being when he was thrown off a train in South Africa. Harry Bernstein became a celebrated writer at the age of 98.

I suggest that, whatever *form* the expression of our life purpose takes—whether to lead a movement to free a nation, create works of art, build a community or a giant corporation, create a family, or simply quietly and humbly go about being ourselves—each share a common *essence*: creativity and a contribution to the whole that only we, following our life path, inclinations, tendencies, and persistent desires, could possibly make. In this way, the question of our life purpose is a simple one, with no striving or struggle necessary. Our life purpose is a natural consequence of our being who we are. In discovering our authenticity and living from this realization a clarity of vision emerges from the infinity of possibilities. Opportunities, connections, and synchronicities are magnetized into our experience, allowing the form to take shape. The commonality of creating and contributing is due to our being, in essence, a spark of the divine flame, which we might characterize as creative Love. The human journey is about discovering how we can, each of us in our unique way, express this. How can we bring forth our deepest essence into the world? By being our deepest essence. Now.

In a world so disconnected from the truth of our unity, we can see it is necessary for our collective well-being that we recognize that living our life's purpose is a very impersonal personal matter. To live fully, joyously, and authentically is the life of an evolutionary.

At once, failure is impossible, a concept created by fear, itself an illusion of a mind that has momentarily forgotten only Love is real.

What have you always dreamed of?
What is most important to you?
What is your greatest passion?

I asked these questions of a friend at dinner one evening. Her first response was that her dream was to watch her favorite television programs and chill—nothing grand like my aspirations or those of our friends, she added. Without prompting, as a sort of "by the way," she then went on to reveal that building an orphanage and caring for uncared-for children had *always* been her greatest dream, and what she desired above all else. She went on to explain that she had supported her husband when he gave up his well-paid job in order to create a business providing affordable organic food, an expression of *his* life's purpose. She was hoping this would ultimately lead to the creation of the funds that would make her dream of an orphanage a reality. Let us be bold and free from cynicism or playing small!

In doing so, both my friend and her husband are willing to give up well-paid, successful, safe, and reliable careers in order to express their life's purpose. I have no doubt they will both succeed. For when we touch that within us that we care about more than anything, we access unseen forces that will propel, guide, and inspire us to its fruition. We need only to bring this vision forth into our minds and be prepared to overcome our fears of the unknown and not being "enough." In doing so we transcend the conditioned mind and blaze the way for others. As my friend did, look beyond the easy answer … the answer that our ego and the egos of others might be most comfortable with. What vision, what possibility fills you with joy and inspiration? Who do you need to be for this to become real in your experience?

Why Would We Not Be Living Our Purpose Already?

Why did my friend, a deeply intelligent and caring woman, first downplay her dream? What prevented it from being at the forefront of her mind? Why would we do anything other than singing such a glorious song from the rooftops?

From our fear we are dismissive of the true and beautiful. From our identification with the separate self, we become cynical to mask our fear and insecurity. Within this fear of not being enough, we seek to protect ourselves by being "right" and dismissing anything that might expose our fear or prove us wrong. The remedy, as in all things, is to return our being to Love. Our primary purpose is always a matter of how we are being.

A reaction to the dreamers of a new world, based on

the false premise that there is an objective reality apart from our dreaming is to "be realistic" ... to keep in mind that ideas of Love and Truth are all well and good, but "*in reality*," they are too idealistic to be of much value. Such talk is ignorant of a scientific discovery so epic that over one-hundred years on we are still integrating it into our worldview. This discovery is that reality is not the fixed, solid, material world our senses perceive. At its most fundamental level it is a collectively co-created fluid in constant motion. Each time we offer an opinion on the world—what it is, what it could be, and what it cannot be—we are voting. Life is inherently democratic. Whereas it may appear that the ideal of political democracy representing the needs and interests of the people has degenerated to a few vested interests looking after themselves, "life democracy" is alive and well.

We are in each moment casting our votes via our thoughts, intentions, feelings, and actions. We are in each moment part of the "problem" or part of the "solution." We can moan about what is wrong, and in that moment be a part of it. If we are imagining only the problem, we are part of it. The moment we imagine the solution, we become part of it. Being our authentic joyful, creative selves, listening to the Love that we are and acting from this being, we are vessels by which evolutionary potential may express through us. Happily millions of us are merrily birthing a new world. This process has been going on for millennia, is peaking in our time, and will inevitably succeed. We can relax and enjoy the ride, taking our seats as creative beings. We are in a stage akin to the caterpillar dissolving in its own acidic juice; there is discomfort and disorientation, we can fail in fear to recognize this is progress and the outcome is assured. Yet this too is the evolving of trust in Love.

Paul Hawken's book *Blessed Unrest* brilliantly and encouragingly elucidates how upwards of two million grass-roots organizations are busy birthing a new world. Of course, don't expect to see this on the TV news. Watch one nightly broadcast and you have watched them all; give your priceless attention to that which brings you joy. Keep in mind that our collective shift occurs just as personal shifts occur—not by attacking that which we seek to change, but by nourishing that which we seek to be and become. When we choose to indulge in thoughts, feelings, and behaviors that are more fun than those that dominate our old operating system, we naturally fuel a movement towards this new way of being. And when we make habitual a new way of being, the old one dies by its obsolescence.

Following this reasoning, I never sought to battle depression, addictions, or indeed cancer. Rather, I have sought to create a new, greater order of harmony in which there would not be a place for any of the old dysfunctions. What we resist persists. In loving and allowing, our heart's desires blossom. We will discover that rising to a new level of thinking, feeling, and being is the only way we will see the old become history. The old does not make way for the new; rather, it will battle for its life. The new becomes the new by *being*.

Life's Purpose

Ultimately it becomes clear that our life's purpose is Life's purpose. Through living our own life's purpose, committed to our deepest dreams and passions, in touch with our true being, characterized by joy, we become an expression of Life's purpose. We access and express a power which births universes.

I find it curious that, in our Western culture, we use the words *idealistic* and *idealism*—meaning "the belief in or pursuit of ideals"—in a pejorative sense. What are we saying to ourselves, about ourselves, when we dismiss talk of peace and love as being idealistic and *something to be discouraged*? What world would we be living in without our idealists? Everything good, true, and beautiful comes from the belief in and pursuit of ideals. And we dismiss such a pursuit as being "unrealistic." *That's the whole point!* We are seeking to create something that is not currently real in form, yet we know exists in our hearts. Let us be idealists, loud and proud. Let us be unrealistic until reality is rather more functional!

Let us heed Irish playwright George Bernard Shaw's assertion that "The reasonable man adapts himself to the world; the unreasonable one persists in trying to adapt the world to himself. Therefore, all progress depends on the unreasonable man." Is it time for more men (and women, of course) to be unreasonable in what we see as possible for ourselves and for humanity?

Whether we are looking to live our life's purpose purely for our own well-being (which increases the well-being of the whole) or purely for the well-being of the whole (which increases our well-being), we are called to be idealists and to give more than the fearful cynicism which so often passes for intelligent comment.

The Purpose of My Life

My life's purpose is to *be* a source of love and truth by whatever means possible. This is a moment-to-moment practice, each moment a meeting to be conducted with love. This is true whether other humans are present or not, and especially so when they are. In terms of form, I choose writing, coaching, speaking, leading workshops, building companies, and communities ... and remaining open to whatever encourages dropping any of these and pick up another pursuit as an expression of this being.

How do I know this is my life's purpose? Because when I am living it, such as writing these words now, I am consumed by it, I experience joy, and I come alive. The first time I delivered a presentation about love and truth, how to suffer less and be in joy more, I felt as if I had come home. I know when I am living my life's purpose because I feel great. If I am regularly not feeling good, I need to reassess my current path.

Let it be clear: living our life's purpose, once we have hacked through the thickets of our fear and procrastination, is fun and need not involve struggle. The more we allow ourselves to be consumed in our purpose, the more effortless it becomes. The moments of pain, anguish, and anxiety fly by all the faster, whilst the contentment lingers longer. We learn to recognize the inevitable challenges and difficulties of creation as opportunities for growth, invitations to reaffirm what is important now.

When we begin to live our life's purpose, our burning love overcomes our fears and dissolves our cynicism. In the process, we gain a life that is so very worth living. Indeed, those who are living their purpose are inspired to share their experiences and make clear the nature of their endeavors and inspire others. For there is no sham drudgery here, no struggle, no obligation other than to one's own inner being. There is an effortless, exalted state of ever more subtle gradations of delighted contentment. There is the inner state of heaven to be found here on Earth when we live our lives as their grandest expression, in service of Earth, humanity, and our grandest ideals. There is good reason to search for 'something more'. And there is good reason, when we begin to find it, to give our lives to it.

If you are searching for your purpose, remember you already have it. It's inside you now. Become still and listen; allow it to be heard. Fret not at what form it will take—astronaut, beekeeper, president, or conscientious parent … or all four. As you identify the guiding principles, the being of it and committed to living it, you will be guided step by step. If you are like me, you will probably forget, only to remember more deeply. Be patient. All happens in its own good time.

It is also true that every moment, every thought, every feeling, every action is a vote. We are either in love or fear, in unity or separation, in joy or despair. We are either being the new consciousness seeking to emerge through us, or perpetuating that which is dying and suffering the stuffy smell of unlived life. We are either progressing in the living of our life's purpose or we are not. We are either having fun or enduring its absence.

Time, were it to exist, would wait for no one. So, what is important now?

Questions for Altering Reality

- *What is your grandest dream? If you knew that you could create whatever circumstance in life you could, that would bring you the greatest lasting joy and fulfillment, what would your life look like? How would it make you feel?*
- *What beliefs and decisions have you previously allowed that have prevented you from pursuing this dream?*
- *What beliefs and decisions will support you in living your life's purpose, your life of the greatest possible joy, contribution, and contentment?*

*Whatever a person's mind dwells
on intensely and with firm resolve,
that is exactly what he becomes.*

—The Buddha

*Each of us makes the epoch in which
we live.*

—Carl Jung

Chapter 6:
The Gift of Co-Creativity

Why Me?

It was a couple of months post diagnosis, and one of my most intelligent and perspicacious friends made a comment that was removed from my experience. It helped clarify how and why this experience of being diagnosed with a life-threatening illness was unfolding for me personally in much the same manner (with great curiosity) and emotional content (great excitement) as a trip to the zoo.

He said, "You must constantly be asking yourself, 'Why me?'"

The truth was that even the idea of asking such a question had not occurred to me until that moment. It was a laughable notion, particularly in the elevated state of consciousness I was in at the time. Such a self-centered stance appeared so obviously unproductive. I might have responded, "Why would I want to ask that?"

The questions we ask, and how we ask them, are powerful determinants of our experience. Earlier in my life I had several times asked "Why me?" upon finding myself in different places of self-pity, yet had only experienced its undesirable consequence. As a teenager I had at times assumed that, in my current position in life, I was somehow a victim of life's vicissitudes, that my sufferings and challenges were unique and of a different order to those of others. I would label this common attitude "poor little me" or the "victim level of consciousness." From your own experiences, you may have noticed that this position is not much fun. We can learn to live beyond it to live a full life.

I recall well the moment, as a twenty-one-year-old, when I realized how *extraordinarily* lucky I was. I saw how the bare facts of my existence—being white, English, and male—made life easier for me than for many others. I had my sister and parents and the love they gave me in my formative years, an extraordinary blessing. I had a top education, a body that was generally fit and functional, a countenance that was typically regarded as being better than ugly, the extraordinary meetings with key people at key times, and the teachers at my school who prevented much difficulty by successfully campaigning against those who wanted me expelled. It was a humbling epiphany.

The clarity and depth of this realization exposed the underlying meta-narrative of my life up until that point as inaccurate. Whilst many more of these moments were required to begin to learn some basic humility, this first revelation created a seismic shift in how I viewed the world and my place in it. I realized how profoundly lucky I was, and I became more and more grateful. This is not to say my new state of being was not punctuated with dips into the old state, and into depressions of huge magnitude in which I felt the depths of worthlessness and hopelessness. I can characterize this revelation, however, as the first political scandal in which my old self's story had been exposed in all its tawdry, narcissistic glory, and its position clearly demonstrated to be untenable.

That the "poor little me" persona would—and occasionally still does—seek to reassert its power is just part of the process of being human: the spiraling nature of human development whereby we forever revisit the same themes from different vantage points. "We have a thousand selves," said German–Swiss writer and painter Hermann Hesse. "I am multitudes," wrote American poet Walt Whitman. The sooner one allows the complexity of this contradiction, and fully embraces its reality in personal experience, the sooner simplicity and harmony of being can emerge.

Having identified myself as extraordinarily lucky, I was fascinated to observe the effect that this realization had on my life. In short, I seemed to get demonstrably luckier, and so my life became a virtuous circle of ascending degrees of luckiness, both in feeling and in experience, the one feeding back into the other. Realizing one's luck is an eloquent and effective response to the vicious, negative vortex we create when we tell a story that life is difficult, unkind, or unfair, or when we indulge in any other particular expression of self-pity.

Whenever we experience events congruent with the

dominant focus of our narrative, we are prone to interpret this as evidence of the story's truth and justification for continuing to tell the story. All stories and prophesies have the potential to be self-fulfilling if there is sufficient belief and sustained attention. What you focus on, you will manifest. Therefore, choose your story carefully. Become conscious of your story, especially your meta-narrative, your most cherished beliefs, the story underscoring your life.

Notice that your meta-narrative was formed by the mind of a younger you, combined with anonymous hand-me-downs from the collective soup. Question to what degree these conditioned beliefs are in harmony with what you now know and what you wish your life experience to be, and possibly for the first time actually *choose* a story. Naturally you will pick one that's fun to tell and has a happy ending. Unless you don't, of course, for as is clearly evident in the world around us, it's always possible to choose to be disempowered, to choose to evade responsibility for one's life experience, and even to choose misery and death.

Shifting my most common question in life from "Why me?" to "How lucky am I?" was initially jarring. It happened in stages. The self-pitying "Why me?" shifted first into the guilt-laced variant, "Why am I so lucky when others suffer so?" Eventually, a more joy-filled, open-hearted recognition of my good fortune naturally emerged, and the question became, "How can I help others be more lucky?"

Quite clearly, in any event and circumstance, the

question "Why me?" makes as much sense as asking, "Why *not* me?" It is, in its typical victim mode, an unanswerable question that is but a reflection of one's tone of mind at the time and not a genuine enquiry that seeks for true understanding.

After my friend brought the question to mind, I realized that I actually had asked it, only in quite a different way. It was really an echo of the "Why am I so lucky?" question I had installed many years back. Before surgery and the upgraded diagnosis I could point to the good luck that the brain tumor was benign. Following the more precise diagnosis post-surgery, I focused on it being treatable, on it being one of the better types of a stage three, on the gift of my having access to a talented and dedicated transformational team of neurosurgeons, masseurs, energy healers, naturopaths, coaches, and teachers that I could afford to engage, and even on the gift of my still being alive after a couple of months. And, oh yes, the fact that, not in spite of, but *because* of the diagnosis, I was having the time of my life, touching greater depths of joy and revealing a capacity to transform despair than I had ever imagined possible.

So, yes, "Why me?" is a question I might now ask in such a way as to remind myself of the answer, which is, hopefully you are beginning to see, the story I have been programming my mind with for many years: "Because I am an extraordinarily lucky person!" The events of the last years have bestowed a further depth of realization to the nature of the world: this lucky guy finds himself living in a world of infinite intelligence and mystery that somehow seems set up to facilitate his growth and evolution into ever higher spheres of wisdom, love, joy, service, and co-creative capacity!

And so I ask, smiling into the silence, "How lucky am I?"

Self-Diagnosis

I recall sharing with people in the first weeks after the diagnosis that I had brain *cancer*. It seemed to have a gravitas that my experience of "having a brain *tumor*" did not possess. I once liked a bit of drama, especially to provoke a response, and I have been prone to exaggerate (unconsciously) in order to make a point. The point I sought to make was that it is possible to smile in the face of death; it is possible to encourage and to be happy regardless of circumstance.

The words *brain cancer* possess such oomph, and are so often associated with death, that, of course, for very good reason, they appear actually not to be used much. Therefore, whilst, if you have a tumor on your liver or lung, for example, you are said to have "X cancer," in the medical circles I moved in, it's always termed a *brain tumor* rather than *brain cancer*. It might be said that *brain tumor* is indicative of the type of tumor, cancer being reserved only for aggressive tumors. However, this was the language I noticed being used from the outset, even when this point had not yet been clarified following the initial MRIs that suggested a benign tumor.

I hope this suggests a creeping understanding within conventional medicine of how important language is—for language has associations and implications that create real-time biochemical/physical effects. The relatively young field of psychoneuroimmunology evidences that the emotions and feelings generated by the stories we tell affect the functioning of our immune systems. We can see that the patient's expectations and beliefs—and thus the prognosis and doctor's manner—are causative factors in health outcomes.

Aware of this from previous research, I chose my own prognosis, which I typed, printed, and laminated for reference: "The brain tumor was a gift from my soul, from Spirit, inviting me to heal my wounds, to bring love and light into every corner of my being, and to live my life as the expression of the joy and wisdom that I am. I accepted the invitation, and through healing my brain, I deepened my skills and knowledge of healing and transformation. I now live a life of abundance, traveling the world, guiding and inspiring others in the service of their healing and awakening. I live in joy, in conscious creation, in appreciation, and possibility. I know I am loved."

You will note I wrote this in the present tense, with the outcome already having happened, so on reading it my mind experienced the outcome as real now. Similarly professional sports people have long used the power of visualizing the race or event and the preferred outcome. Experiments have demonstrated that *only imagining* muscle growth (in a regular and focused fashion) is sufficient to create measurable growth relative to control groups over the same period. The groundbreaking work of the Simontons in the 1970s demonstrated such mind power can be applied to reducing tumor mass through visualization alone. Interestingly, my metaphysics when I wrote the self-diagnosis included no real concept of a soul or Spirit, yet these are the words I used. One could as easily replace them each with "Life" to create a similar effect.

This is the story I chose to live, and whilst the route including surgery and radiotherapy was not part of the plan, I am happy to surrender the details to Spirit.

Thinking *is* Magical

Any sufficiently advanced technology
is indistinguishable from magic.
—*Arthur C Clarke*

Could our own minds, be the technology that will, when more fully understood and potentiated, revolutionize our world? It is old news that the human mind is creative by nature. As the Buddha is recorded in the Dhammapada, "We are what we think," and, as the Bible states, "As he thinks in his heart, so is he" (Proverbs 23:7). We live in a culture that still believes mind and matter to be separate. In addition its institutions are motivated to condition individuals to believe themselves powerless. The ego can find this lack of personal responsibility alluring and so will typically accept the conditioning. In these ways resistance to a full embrace of the mind's power continues. However, owing to the mind's power, the more we believe our minds to be powerfully creative, the more we experience life utilizing this creative power, and vice versa. We can rely on personal experiential enquiry alone, but there is no leap of faith required here. Scientific evidence from many fields of research—neurocardiology, epigenetics, parapsychology, and, some argue, quantum mechanics—supports the mind's causative role. Perhaps most exciting is the evidence that our thoughts and emotions affect gene expression.

Despite the scientific evidence, belief in the mind's power can be dismissed as "magical thinking." Such a response is predictable because such "new" perspectives challenge people's existing belief systems (which many prefer not to update) and, if embraced, require a fundamental shift in how we engage with reality. This shift, I would suggest, is nothing less than *the* shift that we as a collective mind are in the throes of bringing into being. The shift is from living as a separate, disempowered "I" in a world perceived as primarily physical, to realizing we are highly interdependent and interconnected being—more "we" than "I"—living in a world we know to be primarily immaterial and with which we are in constant, complex, *creative* exchange.

One might notice the huge level of personal responsibility the second worldview engenders. Clearly, in a society in which many believe they are powerless and live primarily as *consumers*, this new worldview is unlikely to immediately grip the mainstream. Of course such shifts throw up opposition. This is the nature of change. As the German philosopher Arthur Schopenhauer put it: "All truth passes through three stages. First, it is ridiculed. Second, it is violently opposed. Third, it is accepted as being self-evident."

I can see much of this collective process at work in my personal enquiry into how life works. What once would have seemed ridiculous is now self-evident. It is helpful to keep in mind why and how such criticisms arise as we seek to arrive at our own understanding as free as possible from the biases and beliefs of the age in which we live.

Having looked at the inevitability of resistance to any new ways of viewing the world—and keeping in mind that resistance will equally face nonsense as well as new levels of understanding—let's offer some context for why the notion that our minds directly influence physical reality is especially problematic. Such a view is heavily dependent on a crumbling edifice of Western thought; namely, that mind and matter are two distinct entities separate from one another in their functioning.

Traditional materialist views offered no framework by which we could explain how thoughts and feelings in themselves might influence matter other than through known mechanistic laws. Candace Pert's book *Molecules of Emotion* on the science behind mind–body medicine is one of many to have shed light on how our feelings have biochemical correlations within our own body. Science increasingly points to a unity of the immaterial and material. The mind's power is only "magical" (in the sense of unrealistic and unbelievable) if we assume the mind and the physical world to be truly separate in essence and substance. When we realize the two to be, in a more fundamental sense, one, it is easy to see how what might have been seen as magic and miracles are merely part of a magical-and-miracle-orientated mind.

Of course this all becomes most persuasive when seen through direct experience, typically as a result of some form of spiritual practice. If you have not yet found the time to meditate for a few thousand hours, or been lucky enough to be graced with the gift of spontaneous unitive consciousness, I suggest that the same conclusion of the unitive nature of reality can be reached through a study of those who claim they *have*—the numerous sages, saints, and mystics of history, who, indeed, offer close to a unanimity of accounts across time and place.

Just as effectively, through an open-minded study of the scientific data, one may come to a similar conclusion. If you take this path, I would advise you first to become familiar with not only the methodology but the philosophy and history of science, apply what you learn to the current beliefs and biases, look to the edges of scientific discovery, and remember that just because a lot of scientists agree on something, it isn't necessarily scientific!

Defining what is, is always—every moment and every word—a two-way street. More primary and important than the doctor's diagnosis is the meaning you make of it. Studies of the "nocebo effect" give examples of how patients often conform to doctors' diagnoses; for example, dying as predicted by a cancer diagnosis, even when it is later discovered that the person did not, in fact, have cancer; realizing tumor mass reduction by a radiation machine later found not to have been working; or dying exactly within the time frame of the doctor's prognosis (six months to the day!). I recommend physician Lissa Rankin's excellent recent work for an exploration of this topic as it applies to health from a Western doctor's perspective.

Doctors have to meet the considerable challenge of giving accurate and "realistic" information (potentially as determined by a court of law) whilst hopefully being aware that the tone of their communication that suggests optimistic or pessimistic interpretation of the data is one of many causative factors in their patient's health. As patients we must be mindful to be as free as possible of the limiting beliefs and well-intentioned ignorance of others, whether doctors or family members, and be willing to take 100% responsibility for our health.

It is easy to be swayed by the herd. I recall watching a Louis Theroux documentary on British television (BBC) in 2014. In this particular episode of *LA Stories*, cameras followed three or four individuals during their healthcare experience in Los Angeles. The thrust of the show was to question the wisdom of keeping people alive when quality of life was seemingly minimal, such as people in permanent vegetative states, or of providing expensive and very painful treatments to cancer patients with poor prognoses. However, the program threw up a surprise via a case at Cedars-Sinai Medical Center. A young man had been admitted in a comatose state with likely brain damage from a drug overdose. After 72 hours he was still unresponsive, and the prognosis was very bleak. A neurologist looked at the scans and concluded that in the unlikely event of the man waking up he would be in a permanent vegetative state. The case doctor tried to break the news to the family that there was no hope. They insisted, his sister in particular, with a curious certainty, that, whilst they understood the doctor's position, they did not accept it and he would wake up. I confess to thinking them naive, unable to accept the tragic truth. Yet, after 17 days, this man woke up. Not only that, he could speak and was soon walking. On expressing his delighted surprise to the sister, Theroux received a curt "I told you!" as if to question how anyone could have ever doubted. This was an exceptional case. However, it brings credence to the notion one integrative doctor shared with me that, knowing what we know about the mind (and the more common than we might perceive "miracle cases"), there is no such thing as "false" hope. Our challenge is to balance an embrace of all outcomes with holding a particular one in mind; to surrender and actively utilize the mind's creative power at once.

Earlier in this chapter I mentioned the curious use of language surrounding the tumor. There was a particular instance with my neurosurgical team that demonstrated just how arbitrary the language of diagnosis can be. Having rather curiously started to use the term *brain cancer*, I asked my neurosurgeon if my condition was indeed cancer rather than "just" a tumor. A report of his had stated it was a "benign malignancy." He replied that yes it was—there was abnormal cell expression and malignant cell growth; thus, it was technically cancer. However, later that same day my neurological nurse specialist said during a phone conversation, "Of course you don't have cancer, yet if it were to develop ..." So in the same day my medical team told me I did and then did not have cancer; perhaps the quickest spontaneous remission on record? I remember finding this rather funny, and I was happy to dwell in the ambiguity and focus on the one bit of medical data that was unequivocally important: is the tumor growing or not? First being aware of physical reality as it currently appears may be important if we seek to adjust it; to think otherwise would indeed be magical!

This incident and many others demonstrated to me that, even within the world of medical science, which we tend to characterize as highly precise with considerable degrees of certainty, there are heaps of "gray areas" and mountains of "don't knows." I am deeply grateful that the majority of my medical professionals were open and honest about this lack of understanding and answered many of my questions about the nature of the tumor with a simple "I don't know."

Some criticism of "magical thinking" is valid; for example, there is not always an easy fix to life's challenges, and changing our thinking by itself may be insufficient. Changing what we *do* is clearly significant. However, what is truly required in order to change outer experience is to change our entire *being*. This includes feelings, beliefs, choices, and unconscious thought processes. This does, of course, starts with our thinking. Popular expressions of the law of attraction typically do not clearly explain that this is a lifelong journey that requires inner work at considerable depth and subtlety. It is true transformation, and it is but a choice away. It happens now, because in every moment "self" and "world" die and are reborn. Yet it is also true that patience and persistence are prerequisites to seeing a consistently different self and world. We pay attention to our inner world, realizing its primacy, while believing the physical reality to be very real. And we act accordingly. It is one thing to know that matter is 99.99999 percent empty and responsive to mind; it is another to be aware of this each moment and be capable of performing miracles. Until we have mastered walking through walls, we use the doorway!

How doctors term the situation in my brain is of course not irrelevant. However, they generally possess a limited understanding of what is going on at a physical level, let alone on more subtle levels of reality. Thus I remain grateful for their skills and capacities and the intention to serve whilst at once being aware of the limitations of what they offer. Having had the formative nature of the story I tell about life demonstrated time and time again, I am careful about what I take to be true and thus hold in my mind. I have received and accepted the gift of co-creativity.

There is one gift left to explore, the greatest of them all.

Questions for Altering Reality

- *Has the time come for you to adjust a story you tell about yourself or about life itself?*
- *What is the most inspiring story of your life you can tell and live into?*
- *Which thoughts and beliefs that you see arise as you read this chapter are supportive of your well-being? Which thoughts and beliefs are not supportive of your well-being? And what limiting beliefs is it time to discard?*

Rather than money, than fame,
give me truth.

—Henry David Thoreau

You want the truth?!
You can't handle the truth!

—Jack Nicholson playing Col. Nathan R.
Jessup to Tom Cruise's Lt. Daniel Kaffee
in A Few Good Men

Truth can only be experienced.

—A Course in Miracles

Chapter 7:
The Gift of Oneness

This last gift cannot be spoken of. Yet what but the ineffable is truly worthy of words?

This gift is worth being born and dying for. It is the greatest gift I have ever received yet I already had it. To speak of it as an experience wrongly implies beginning or end; placing it in time denies its timelessness. Even speaking of "it" we are prone to suffer the pretence that it is something other than what we are, enduring the arrogance that we could somehow be apart from Life itself. What could a flame say of fire?! To speak of it in terms of being given to me is relatively true, yet so preposterously partial, as to require a new language be learnt.

This language is silence. Yet I if I am to write this book (and golly I have tried not doing so!) this is the one topic that must be covered, for it includes, informs, and inspires all that is. Nothing makes sense without it; it is how I was *blessed* with a brain tumor. In its remembrance, no questions remain. It is the culmination of a life-long quest and at once the beginning of a new chapter of spiritual life.

It is the deepest and most prolonged experience of the state of non-dual consciousness of my life. It is the gift of Oneness.

Altered States of Consciousness

Our normal waking consciousness, rational consciousness as we call it, is but one special type of consciousness, whilst all about it, parted from it by the filmiest of screens, there lie potential forms of consciousness entirely different. We may go through life without suspecting their existence; but apply the requisite stimulus, and at a touch they are there in all their completeness.
—William James

As a teenager I would experience the most curious moments when all that I knew, including my sense of self, would fall away completely. I would be walking along and suddenly all knowledge of who I was, where I was, even *what* I was would disappear. It might sound like a disconcerting experience; however, there was no one to be disconcerted because the structure of my mind that *does* disconcerted was momentarily offline.

These experiences were wonderful, inherently perfect, and deeply peaceful. Then, curiosity would kick in and there would be a questioning: "What is this? Who am I?" and the manifestation of a *me* would slowly re-emerge. "Ah yes, I am me. I am Will Pye. It's 2:30

on a Thursday, and this is Cambridge." Reality and normality would resume.

At the time, I simply thought it was a very interesting experience. I did not share it with anyone because it sounded a bit weird. I was at an age where I wanted to appear normal, as this seemed to be a prerequisite for having friends. I have since learned that to be "normal" in this mad world is about as poor a comment on intelligence and sensitivity as exists.

What can I now say was happening to my young self in those moments of disappearance? The self-experience was interrupted, yet something remained. Awareness itself. This awareness. The awareness within which this reading, this writing, all ideas of you and of me arise. The typical object/subject split of conventional consciousness would cease, and there would be just *this* "awarenessing." This, and all that is arising within this, is *oneness*.

This may seem like an extraordinary experience, yet following thousands of hours of meditation practice I see now that what was happening was merely what is happening all the time, moment after moment. These instances were seemingly "stretched" so as to make it more noticeable that this "me" had ceased to be. This seemed to be easy for the younger mind to internalize. The more investment in creating our story of self, the more conditioning obstructs seeing that who we think we are does not exist, other than as a construct in thought. Thus as we grow up and internalize the norms and assumptions of our culture, such glimpses of our true nature may be pathologized as dysfunctions of the mind. If we are lucky, they are interpreted as "mystical experiences." Caught up in sustaining the story of "me" we interpret the moments of seeing clearly as exotic and thus distant, labeling the experience as "spiritual awakening," something that happens to only a select few. In such a way, in lives typically unexamined, identification with the ego sustains itself. We think enlightenment, like death, happens only to other people. Yet enlightened mind is ubiquitous, and is reading these words right now.

The Greatest Gift of All: Oneness as Personal Experience.

The *realization* of impermanence—that all is in flux, ever-changing, and nothing lasts, specifically me—is indeed a rare jewel. It is not mere folly that Tibetan monks meditate beside corpses to break through the psychological trick through which our personal identity is experienced as ongoing.

In facing and embracing death, I cast aside all plans, dreams, fears, ambitions, anxieties, desires, and ideas of who I should or should not become. In short, I cast aside *me*. I let go of all I thought I was. So, what happens when what we think we are is released? What happens as a consequence of surrender?

What happens is that we realize what we are. A *realization* of the truth of oneness is certainly the greatest gift of this unfolding. It is the experience rather than the idea that is most challenging to express. English is an especially dualistic language, its grammatical structure insisting upon a subject and an object. Apparently, Japanese and many of the languages of the Native Americans are far less grammatically dual. English is a perfect language for commerce and science, but has its limitations for describing reality. Its structure, of course, reflects and informs conventional thinking and typical experience—there is, it seems, you and me, this and that. In addition to the insistence on subject and object, English requires every event be placed in time, which we call, appropriately enough, a "tense." However, the experience of awakening to the truth of what we are is timeless; it occurs outside time. With the reactive ego and its obsessive fearful planning and rehashing of the past set aside, there is just this glorious moment, utterly perfect, resplendent, needing nothing. What a relief!

Once I discarded the self-structure, what was left was boundless presence. Looking at the world around me, I noticed there was nothing keeping that which was seeing separate from that which was being seen. Images of common objects, such as a table or tree, would of course form; however, I was not apart from them. There was a fluidity to perception; it made as much sense to say "I am the table" as it did to say "The table is over there." The same was true of people. There being no separate self in experience means just that—there is no other to project on to another body, just as there is momentarily none within the seeing. We truly see the world and all its inhabitants as we are; when we are in touch with our own loving presence, we detect this same quality in others. This allows a delicious intimacy to exist when encountering another human being. The extraordinary beauty and radiance of each person is clear to see.

The world took on a sparkling luminescence, a radiance that made *everything* wonderful. No distinction was made between that which we would normally distinguish as beautiful or ugly, valuable or worthless. Every little detail of everything was astonishing just in its being; nothing had changed, yet all was completely different. There was a tremendous lightness in each moment; there was nothing to be taken seriously, no problems could possibly be imagined. "Problems" require thought and identification. Beyond both there is just stuff to do, situations to respond to. This took some getting used to and created the occasional amusing incident such as when someone told me their grandmother had died. Reveling in being, adjusting to this freshness yet still with a conditioned movement to say something, "Wonderful" fell from my lips. This was no problem and a one-off; I saw that often a simple nod might be best. Being in a state of peace and causeless joy is very unusual by the norms of our culture.

"Me" appeared absent for a while, but thankfully not entirely dissolved. When it arose—"it" being the personality structure, the voice we identify with, the thoughts, feelings, and memories we aggregate into our self— it was an it, rather than me. This was so very delightful because when one is only the object of awareness there is no scope for reactivity. Or rather if there is reactivity it is seen and no action is taken. Much time was spent laughing at this character, so clueless, so insane with its wanting, scheming, and so on, oblivious to the fact of its very limited reality. For all its foolery, it was clearly utterly harmless, so long as it was seen through. Indeed the ego has some important functions.

One of these functions consists of maintaining our physical life, and in deciding I was going to create a self-induced healing there was a seemingly necessary interruption in the bliss. There now existed an albeit gently held future-orientated success (self-induced healing completed) and failure story (tumor still there). I had ceased to surrender fully; I wanted to be in control. It was nothing less than miraculous and awe-inspiring to witness the vast expanse of pure being, contract into this identity, and be so convincing. There was no sense of regression or this being undesirable, just fascinating phenomena, just perfection unfolding. Only ego finds ego undesirable. I would certainly rediscover this in less enlightened moments following those giddy first few months. I have come to realize this return into identification was a necessary part of the process of awakening.

When I "failed" and embraced the use of surgery and radiotherapy, I found further opportunity to surrender my attachment to a particular route to healing. I began to learn to balance desiring certain creations, such as to be healthy, and surrendering attachment to a particular route and letting go of the result itself. In this state, desiring, creating, and the joy of imagining delightful phenomena and experiences are embraced and their manifestation realized now. Energetically this is very different from hoping for something to happen but actually being in lack or fear. If we want to experience abundance, health, and happiness, we simply experience abundance, health, and happiness. When this is our consistent inner experience, this is our consistent outer experience. For "inner" and "outer" are, like psychological time and the ego, constructs of thought, useful tools for playing the human game, not to be confused with Truth.

So, love and deeply respect the ego. If there is an absence of self-love there is identification with ego; if there is judgment, of anything, there is ego present. The paradox is that the ego is tricky, slippery, and guileful, and it will do everything to maintain identification, including using self-loathing or the belief it is not active (as distinct from the experience of its absence).

An Analogy of Awakening

Soon after the awakening experience I was watching the play *Warhorse* at a London theatre. During the performance, I experienced being detached from the experience, as much watching the audience watching the play as I was watching the play itself. Indeed I was watching myself watching myself watching the audience. I was not immersed in the experience with the requisite suspended disbelief upon which enjoyment depends. In contrast, I could observe this immersion all around me and especially in the big guy in front of me. He was having a great time and was evidently deeply involved in the twists and turns of the plot, so much so that when a goose (represented in the play by a goose-shaped piece of wood mounted on a stick and animated by an actor) *just* failed to make it through a door, he was overcome with excitement and let out an unrestrained "Oooh!" The thought arose that this was a disproportionate response to this little event, irrelevant to the plot.

A pair of realizations crystallized, clearer than ever:

1. Our interaction with life is like a theatregoer's interaction with a play on the stage. All the world is indeed a stage, and we imagine ourselves in many different roles, whereas at a deeper level we are just this watching ... this awareness, at once the theatregoer, the play, the characters, the audience, and that which is witnessing all this. It is like being in a mirrored elevator where we see infinite reflections of the one real being. You and me, and every apparent one, are reflections of the One. Remarkably, somehow, from within the experience of separation, the experience of *being*, as what we are, always present

yet which had somehow escaped our attention, is noticed. We are this ordinary mind, so well hidden from the seeker, in full view. The seeker *is* that being sought.

2. The absolute Truth is that nothing really matters or has any meaning. Thus all "serious" responses to life are disproportionate; when we inevitably experience moments of resistance, we have forgotten we are watching a play. Nothing has any significance beyond that which we give it. Of course to then merely *believe* it is meaningless and live a nihilism is but one story, and not such a fun one. Such a belief is profound insight processed by the ego into a dull philosophy. When we live authentically we *see* that *nothing* matters. Yet, curiously, we care deeply; love or compassion is realized as an essential property of existence. Simultaneously we act, knowing *everything* matters. Where there is no meaning, there is infinite meaning, endless possibility. We learn to be in this world, but not of this world—much as watching a play. More delicious paradox!

This realization that nothing matters does not necessarily mean, either figuratively or literally, that we cease going to the theatre. We continue to play along as an apparently separate being, simultaneously experiencing the oneness we are, ever more deeply realized. We integrate imminence and transcendence. Perhaps this is what is meant when it is said we are created in God's image, for an aspect of the divine, or the Universe if you prefer, is that it is both here and now and beyond us. In maintaining this balance, a divinely human life might be lived. At once we choose the stories to live from and transcend these stories. We play a character we love, and we develop admirable qualities, whilst at the same time realizing the character is a fiction within oneness.

How One is Still One Within Oneness, and the Necessity of Shadow Work

In "enlightenment" the ego is absent, and all that goes with it is absent. It happens in an instant. It is not an experience. It is not an it. Yet, at once, there *is* a process and there are degrees of awakening. The identification with the self-structure does *not* dissolve entirely in the first moment of clarity, apart from in very rare cases, which can be very messy. For most there is a long period when the insight has to be allowed to work its way through the entire being, including the body and the psychology. It is the ultimate paradox and that which leads to endless partiality and confusion in spiritual chat—we are, at once, infinite *and* individuated, impersonal *and* personal. The *experience* is not so confusing, but for dualistic ego thinking, such contradiction is unwieldy, and thus our perspective often ends up in one partiality rather than being able to hold the complexity.

It is vital to embrace this complexity, and for psychological work—*personal* development—to continue post awakening. If this does not happen, the immature psychological structure, through which awakened mind expresses, with aspects still repressed or in "shadow" will express in unconscious and potentially harmful action. We see this in the countless examples of sex, money, or power scandals involving spiritual teachers and their communities. Deep insight, the capacity to drop into non-dual consciousness, what we might call non-identified awareness, is not enough. It only takes a moment of identification to unconsciously express and be destructive. Our capacity for self-deception is huge. Enlightened mind is capable of endless expansion.

Shadow work, bringing into the light the aspects of the individual and collective mind such as fear, greed, and anger that the individual has suppressed or refused to own, is essential for many. If enlightenment is to find full flowering, this must be an ongoing process. Spiritual awakening is not the end of human development, it is its beginning. Indeed, it is far easier to evolve the self-structure when it is seen as an object rather than experienced only subjectively.

As attractive as some end point appears to the ego, as much as we seek a place where never again will we experience pain or loss—an ultimate level of human development—there are certain elements of living with a human body which are inescapable. Enlightenment can be the end of suffering yet also the beginning of feeling our pain more acutely. It is the culmination of a journey and at the same time the beginning of a new stage in our development. So long as we have a body, we have further to go.

An Analogy of Integrating Awakening

Once we have realized we are this vast expanse, that all is perfection unfolding, that the ego is required more to follow than lead, and thought is 90% unnecessary, we might imagine the transition to sitting back and enjoying the perfection unfold to be straightforward. And so it is. Until it's not.

It is rather like the manager (ego) of a factory (your life) who has run the operation for decades only for automated processes to be introduced that are far more effective and efficient. In this new circumstance the manager gets paid the same salary as before, hits bonus automatically every quarter, yet is required to work only a few hours a week in order to open the factory, turn on the machines, and maybe deal with the occasional visitor. They have, on the surface, just as much authority as before. Of course they are delighted—ecstatic! They now have everything they thought they wanted: happiness, freedom, a new level of abundance.

All they really need do is remember the automated systems and trust they will continue to work as they always have.

It is crystal clear, to both the ego manager, the mind or thought, and to the overseer, the "I am" (this pure awareness), that this is progress for all concerned. In theory there should be no resistance. Indeed all is well, and, at first, the manager adjusts to their free time, enjoying being able to give energy to new projects, and to spend more time relaxing, simply being. However, after a few months the manager believes a thought that it shouldn't be this easy and starts spending more time at the factory, needlessly checking on the machines, working forty hours because they always have. This would not be a problem except that the manager's fiddling actually slows down the machines and jeopardizes everyone's well-being. Even though the manager would have claimed to have always desired the shorter hours, the increase in pay, and having more time to explore the world, they refuse to fully let go. Polite reminders to perform the basic tasks and quit the unnecessary meddling go unheeded. At this point the overseer steps in and creates a circumstance that compels the manager to accept their new role. Yet the manager again gets back into the old habits and the cycle continues, leading to situations of greater suffering created to impel the manager to sit back, relax and only act as the situation requires and from joyful inspiration and trust rather than fear or any other integrated emotional charge. This is not a punishment; it is a loving corrective in the best interests of all concerned and of no lasting impact. Such aspects of the process can be helpfully viewed as trials and tribulations, tests if you will, by which the new perspective is integrated more deeply. These tests can be repeated if failed - whilst the period of time spent integrating will vary (at least a decade seems to be average) the outcome is assured. This inevitability is seen with enough time; evolution only moves in one direction, spiraling though it may. With a bit of grace the manager eventually learns to relax and simply enjoy the whir of the machines and delight in witnessing the results of the more integrated operations, playing their part as scripted, and as their heart desires.

Or Is It All Just Brain Dysfunction?

As I was attempting to make sense of all that was being experienced, I encountered an amusing possibility: that perhaps this was not "awakening" but brain dysfunction! Let's consider how our dominant cultural lens, that of materialism, might view my experience. A materialist might first discount my subjective experience, whilst of course not having access to it, and, from within his or her own subjective experience, form a view and claim it to be "objective"! The more lenses the better, so let's enjoy another perspective.

I had encountered Suzanne Segal's story of sudden awakening prior to my diagnosis, yet I later discovered some pertinent details. What I had known before was that she was a mother with no interest in spiritual matters. She then had the experience of personal self-dissolution as she stepped onto a bus in Paris. This example is often cited as evidence that awakening can just happen, without any effort or spiritual practice.

Segal went on, after much confusion and struggle, to make sense of her experience and became a spiritual teacher. The oceanic bliss of her experience became the basis of her teaching, and her story fit in nicely with many a tradition.

However, additional information came to light. After many years, the personal *self* as the locus of consciousness returned, and Segal began to retract some of her teaching. She then became ill, and it was discovered that she had a brain tumor. Speculation amongst sceptics began that the early stages of the tumor might have been the cause of her experience. Her students defended her. Thus, two contradictory perspectives formed. One suggested there was no awakening experience, but rather a phenomenon caused by a dysfunction of the brain. The other view, formed by her students and many who knew her well, was that, contrarily, the tumor was in fact why she began to experience less oceanic bliss and a more egoic identification! Of course one can never know, and I am happy to simply acknowledge both the uncertainty in Segal's case, and also that it is not an unreasonable hypothesis that my own awakening was stimulated by a brain tumor *as distinct from my response to it.*

I would encourage utilizing many lenses—psychological, neuroscientific, philosophical, and subjective—to explore such matters. The possibility that such experiences might be attributed to a tumor rather tickles my sense of humor. I highlight it partly that we remember that all pronouncements on an individual's spiritual attainment, including our own, high or low, is just something we made up, however attached we might be to our teacher or tradition being the greatest or, indeed, to our own lowly non-enlightenedness.

There is very limited neuroscience in the area of awakening experiences, it being hard to coincide an MRI scan and enlightenment. However, there is an increasing volume of studies exploring meditation and the brain, possible links between brain damage and self/other perceptions, mystical experiences, and other "spiritual" attitudes. I came across a summary of such studies in a delightful book *Meditating Selflessly* by James H. Austin, a Zen practitioner of thirty-seven years and professor of neurology, which included a look at the effects of certain brain tumors on religious feeling. The book as a whole details the "ego path" or the parts of the brain that, when operating together with religious feeling, give rise to the experience of *self*. So far as I can tell, and of course I am not trained in this area and can only speculate based on limited study, the location of the tumor I was diagnosed with (upper right parietal) appears to minimize this possibility. Most of the effects reported involve the left-hand part of the brain, a fact illustrated by the famous case of Jill Bolte Taylor, which is detailed in her book *My Stroke of Insight.*

For now I am happy to be amused by even a small possibility that the most profoundly beautiful experience of my life, one that has at once in itself made the whole experience of being alive so much more desirable, and which I would happily die for, is merely the subjective experience of a pathology of neurological functioning!

Given the choice, I think I would go with "spiritual awakening" as the explanation, although, truly, I don't know. Whilst a reductionist scientist and a mystic might find themselves in opposition, especially if each clings to their own view, there is nothing in the views themselves that is inherently oppositional.

Beyond ideas of awakening or brain dysfunction, the only matter of consequence is the degree to which this life is lived with wisdom and compassion. Whatever has or has not happened, am I awake, fully present with all that is, right *now*?

In Part Two we explore how we can all become a little more awake.

Questions for Altering Reality

- *Have you at times noticed aspects of deep freedom and joy in your own experience? What can you do to nurture and encourage such openings? Does the desire to nurture and encourage anything block the experience of freedom and joy available now?*
- *Notice experiencing thoughts, emotions, sensory phenomena, and so on. What is it that is experiencing? Is it a separate "self," the thought "me," or is this a thing which also arises in the experiencing? If you are not what is being noticed, then what are you?!*
- *Whether you have meditated for 10,000 hours*

or never before, for this moment put down all thoughts, wishes, desires, fears, and just be. Maybe take a breath, enjoy the experience of breathing. What do you notice?

When you change the way you look at things, the things you look at will change.

—*Max Planck*

Part Two:
The Seven Invitations

The seven invitations are an opportunity to create the life you desire. Taken together, they represent an upgraded operating system, a new you, and a new life. It might be that there are a few standout invitations that resonate and offer the greatest potential at this time. Explore and, as ever, be your own master, trust your inner guidance.

At the end of each chapter and elsewhere there are suggested integration exercises that will be most impactful if you have a pen and paper handy. Take your time, perhaps explore a chapter a day for a week. In this way, you can fully absorb what you discover. Optimal benefit will occur if you read in a quiet place where you are comfortable and relaxed.

*People are not disturbed by things,
but by the view they take of them.*

—Epictetus

Chapter 8:
It's *All* Opportunity

I have discovered that, with practice, it is possible to see every life event, every circumstance, every pain, discomfort, and "problem" as a gift. And, in looking through this 'lens', that is how they are experienced. Life is more fun this way. I began to see this with hindsight, and now it is clear as circumstances present themselves. When we welcome all of our experiences, life becomes one big opportunity for creative exploration and enjoyment. I have come to regard the "big shit" especially as potential-laden opportunity for growth and discovery. Thus, it is so.

My first great opportunity was the pain and torment of my family breaking up when I was thirteen. In rejecting everything I had learned about life, I began a process to find out what was real for myself. In seeing and experiencing the pain around and within me, I developed compassion. In the intense suffering that arose, I began to learn about skilful and less skilful ways of responding. What originally appeared to be "shit" has been alchemized into the gold of now serving others and witnessing their greater joy and well-being.

The second great opportunity was betraying and losing my first love and creating a pattern of shame and self-loathing. In witnessing my love's hurt, I learned a lesson in responsibility and compassion. In witnessing hurting myself as retaliation, I saw the necessity of forgiveness and being kind and gentle with ourselves as well as others.

The third great opportunity was reaching the nadir of my own personally designed hell and experiencing suicidal despair. I was gifted with the realization that the only way out is to go deeper within. A depth of compassion and willingness to be present with pain was a blessing that I can now share with others. There is no greater kick or high—and I have sampled most—than witnessing yourself serving others.

The fourth great opportunity was facing the compulsive nature of my interactions with marijuana and gambling. This period allowed me to experience great insight into the nature of mind, and compelled me to develop discipline and focus. In experiencing the humiliating pain of disempowerment, I began to learn some humility and what it is to be powerful.

The fifth great opportunity was being diagnosed with a brain tumor. By now there was no time lag in discovering the gift. In realizing this was a gift and opportunity at the outset, I allowed a treasure trove of blessings to be showered upon me, not least of which is the writing of this book.

All this pain has taught me of pleasure; all despair, of joy; self-loathing, of unconditional love; hopelessness, of hope; fear, of trust; suffering, of its cessation; separation, of unity. As I experienced many such opposites, with some extreme polarities, I was presented with the opportunity to discover, in startling luminescence, it's all one.

This dancing with life can be developed with practice. Learning your own moves allows the cessation of problems and suffering. It's worth the effort and worth being patient as we step on our own toes time and time again.

Of course it's easy to experience falling in love, or receive an act of kindness from a stranger, or witness a beautiful sunset, eat a delicious meal, or accept a bouquet of flowers as a gift, and so we begin the dance in these moments, with appreciation. This trains the brain to give emphasis to what is desirable. As we progress, we come to see even the unpleasant and unwanted as a gift. Along the way we might come to such a perspective through noticing often that a "bad" development often turns out to be "good." An example would be that you unexpectedly lose a job yet a couple of months later find yourself earning more money doing what you love. However, ultimately we realize that, even when events transpire that appear not to have a hidden advantage, there is always opportunity to learn and grow, to practice love.

How do we access this gift or opportunity? We choose to look for it. All I need in order to discover the gift or opportunity present in a situation or experience is to view it as such and invite the learning to present itself.

For example, I might feel an intensely uncomfortable emotion. I might wish it weren't there, and notice resistance to it. When I choose to see it as a gift, an intimacy with the circumstance immediately opens up, and the suffering created by the resistance falls away. I am then left with just the emotion. By embracing any circumstance or experience with positive acceptance, we remove the suffering of wishing it were not so and allow all our attention and energy to focus on responding intelligently. Which may simply be to feel what is to be felt.

I might come to learn that this is a chance to allow a part of myself to be integrated. I can embrace the 'bad' feeling as part of experience and love myself all the same. In letting go of resistance, energy can flow freely, I feel less stuck, and space is created for some new potential to manifest. Thus I see that, rather than being a hindrance to my desire to feel good, the bad feeling is an opportunity to deepen my capacity to feel good by allowing pain to arise and fall away and remain as loving presence.

Author Alan Seale elucidates such a perspective with great clarity in "The Four Levels of Engagement." These levels are the lenses we use to view an event and thus determine how we will experience it. Within Seale's beautifully simple model, the first level is "drama," the second is "situation," the third is "choice," and the fourth is "opportunity." In applying these stages to my diagnosis experience, we will see how each might look, what sort of feelings and likely responses they might engender, and how helpful each can be in creating a positive outcome.

Drama

At level one my response is defined by blaming people or circumstances outside myself. I might entertain all manner of thoughts that cause suffering: "This should not be happening!" "Bloody mobile phone companies selling a product that can encourage brain tumors!" "Life is so unfair!" And so on. I might allow the "Why me?" self-pity story to play in my mind. If I do all this, I will undoubtedly not feel so good. I will be creating a stress response of unhelpful hormones in my body. Now I not only have a brain tumor, I have also triggered stress and a retarded immune system.

Situation

At level two I might still feel fear arising, yet I resolve to fix the issue. However, I do so whilst imagining the solution can exist only outside of me. Thus I would give authority away to apparent experts and seek a solution outside of me—a pill or an operation, say—which requires no change on my part. It is not that these options are "wrong," but I am engaging with the issue from a place of disempowerment and thus limiting my options. Feeling powerless and at the mercy of external solutions, as distinct from being at peace with whatever happens, we might suppose there is a mild compromising of my immune system.

Choice

At level three the key distinction is that I first choose how I am going to be. I recognize that it is my stance, or we might say my level of consciousness, which is primary in influencing the experience. I might ask, "Who do I choose to be here? What do I choose as my relationship to my diagnosis? What role do I choose to play going forward?" The actual choice I make in terms of treatment may be no different; however, in choosing who I am being there is a world of difference. I feel empowered, and perhaps there is a mild improvement of my immune system function.

Opportunity

At the fourth level I embrace the circumstance and consider the possibility that there is a gift hidden within these circumstances. I ask, "What's the opportunity here?" This is highly unlikely to be the first time I have employed such a lens with which to view a challenge, and thus I might sense that, as this is quite a big challenge, there is a proportionally bigger opportunity. With this I feel excitement and gratitude, because experience tells me I have never been presented with a challenge I did not have the resources to respond to and ultimately over-come. At this level joy and gratitude create a biochemical response that is supportive of healing; my immune system is significantly *enhanced*.

This briefly outlines the creative process that can occur as we become more aware of how we are being in the world. Our task is to remember to experience this process consciously (and forgive ourselves when we fail). Of course, this is just a model. In experience we might respond at different levels at different times. Twice since diagnosis I responded at the level of situation and from there chose to have surgery, only to change my mind when I recognized this was coming from a place of fear and a desire to have someone else resolve the problem (whilst I bypass the demanding call for transformation). On finally deciding to go ahead with surgery, I could do so knowing I explored all possibilities and seeing the opportunity for a deepening of trust and surrender this choice represented.

Whilst I would not arbitrarily rule out a particular treatment, one option I have ruled out is approaching life with anything but joy and gratitude. The only criterion I have for any treatment decision is that it comes from this deeper wisdom within, from a conscious choice of how I wish to be, and with a consideration of the greatest opportunity on offer. If we notice ourselves engaging at the level of drama or situation, we can see that we would do well to move our perspective volitionally to choice or opportunity and thus create more joy and well-being.

The Opportunity Within Discomfort

I have participated and led many group meditations. A funny thing happens when the leader says "Make yourself comfortable" Most people will move around in their seats, adjusting their posture. We might assume we always want to be sitting comfortably, and yet we often discover, when we look more closely, we are sitting in discomfort.

This serves as a powerful metaphor for how we are prone to live. We forget how important it is to be comfortable in the moment. We forget we only ever experience *this* moment.

We lose clarity amidst ideas of what we think we *should* do—making only others happy or seeking to conform to some idea of being a "good" partner, friend, employee, and so on. We might be lost in the uncomfortable loop of a painful past experience or a feared future.

The good news is that, often, merely a little shuffling of mind and body brings instant comfort.

Happiness is a matter of our personal choice. Try it—can you experience happiness now? This may be as easy as smiling. Notice any resistance—why would you deny yourself happiness in this moment? Just this moment. Recall a happy memory or imagine an event you are looking forward to. Bring a past or future happy event into the present and dwell in it. Another way of changing your emotional state, heart coherence, and neurochemistry in a few seconds is to straighten your posture, open your shoulders a little, and take seven breaths in and out, with the in and out breaths of roughly equal length and no pause between each breath. If this is easy, you can add breathing as if through the center of your chest; breathing in and out of your heart center can increase the positive effects. An advanced step is to ensure breathing abdominally, whilst still focusing on the heart center as the entry/exit point for this breathing.

It is always *now*, and we can always *choose*.

The Opportunity Within Feeling Bad

One of the most startling discoveries I have made, which has been clarified since my diagnosis, is that we can choose emotions. In my experience, emotions are not only phenomena that arise spontaneously—a past hurt seeking to now be felt, owned, and let go—but also modes of experience that I can bring online at will. Some people find it highly profitable to believe that our moods are merely consequences of neurochemistry. Yet it is more truly profitable for the human being when we believe that neurochemistry is a consequence of our mood, which is determined by our attitude, our mental and physical posture. Advances in the understanding of neuroplasticity tell us that a consistently empowered mind literally changes brain physiology. This is crucial information, as studies indicate that antidepressants are no more effective than placebos in 95% of cases of mild to moderate depression.

Studies have shown that holding a horizontal pencil between your teeth for ten minutes a day significantly improves your mood by causing your mouth to take the shape of a smile, which triggers the associated release of "happy" neurochemicals! A sustained particular use of the mind creates lasting change in the physical structure of the brain. Studies have demonstrated this; examples are long-term meditators (who have slightly thicker than average brain linings) and London black cab drivers (in whom the hippocampus enlarges and adapts to help them store a detailed mental map of the city).

Of course, we don't need a pencil to make us smile; neither must we dedicate a lifetime to an activity in order to gain benefits. Mastering our emotions rather than being at their whim is an integral part of our personal and collective evolution. Imagine a world in which there is less unconscious reactivity to anger or fear or greed in business and politics. This world is already unfolding; the old lunacy is becoming more accentuated as part of the process of its falling apart. We catalyze this process by fully integrating in our inner world the changes we wish to observe in the outer world. Each one of us is an incubator for a new world.

Imagine a world in which *you* don't unconsciously react out of your emotional experience. Imagine an emotional mastery that enables choosing your response in any situation. In such a state we naturally choose responses that serve our well-being and do not harm others. We discover we are rather more than faulty machines or selfish animals after all.

Most of us have had the experience of an emotion "happening to" us and of preferring it had not—a sadness arises or a fear struts its stuff. This may be the truth of our experience, and it is not wrong. Sometimes stuff just needs to arise and be felt without resistance. Resisting creates suffering. This process involves no resistance, only acceptance. Within the free flow of acceptance, phenomena naturally and effortlessly change.

We explored volitionally accessing happiness earlier in this chapter. This a good start. However, our natural state is joy, a different category of being altogether. I encourage us to be more ambitious with how we feel. Settling for "fine" or "not bad" is like going hungry at a banquet.

Is it possible to feel joy now?

How about now?

Experiment with this. Maybe if joy seems too lofty, ask "Can I feel okay/content/happy?" first. You might be surprised at how easily and how far you can shift your brain chemistry and mood simply by asking these simple questions.

Such has been my experience in asking "Is joy possible now?" I am often very pleasantly surprised, although less surprised as it becomes the norm, to discover that immediate joy is definitely possible—even if previously I had been feeling a mild despondency.

One particular instance comes to mind that highlights the power of this perspective and exploration. About a year after the diagnosis, the same old despair energy arose—the pain I had spent many years seeking to avoid. I noticed this heavy, dank energy arising, and I felt resistance. I saw sadness over its arising—Ah, not again! With repeated experiments in resistance having failed me, I asked, hesitantly, "Is outrageous joy possible now?" Guess what? It was! The dank energy dissolved, because there was now another show in town ... another character on stage. Joy. How funny this was to observe. All I needed to do was ask! On the journey to this point we will not always find it so simple. However, if we feel voluntary joy to be desirable, we might find it worthwhile to put in the practice.

One such practice is gratitude, which we will explore in Chapter 12.

Beyond Repressing and Expressing

To be crystal clear, I am absolutely not suggesting that any emotion—fear, anger, or sadness—is 'bad' or to be avoided. What I am suggesting is distinct from repressing or denying. What is here is here, and is always most helpfully met with loving and allowing. Whatever it is. It is from this loving and allowing that transformation becomes possible. It is one of the delicious paradoxes we encounter on the path of awakening—we must first embrace that which we wish to transform. Acceptance and transmuting our inner experience are not contradictory; they are different stages of the same process of joy creation. And sometimes we might just settle for being happy with our unhappiness!

Emotions as Information

From a Buddhist perspective, emotional experience is literally a sixth sense. Just as the data from the tongue tell the brain what is being tasted, and the data from the olfactory system offer information on what is being smelled, data related to our emotions purely provide information about what we are feeling. *It's purely information.* There is no drama or story in information; there is no movement to resist or accept in information. It's just data for your perusal. Is that a helpful lens? More helpful than one in which some emotions are good and some bad?

And here is where it gets profoundly simple: if good smells encourage one to hang around the fragrant rose garden or drink that milk because it hasn't gone bad, perhaps good feelings can be used in the same way. If we feel good at work, then keep working. If we feel good walking home down a dark alley, then keep going. If we feel good in someone's company, then keep seeing them. We all do this to some extent; would our lives benefit from using this sense more consciously and consistently?

From this perspective, *depression is useful information.* Indeed, the stronger the depression, the more useful the information; in fact, suicidal despair urges some big shifts in how we operate. Brain chemistry is part of a very helpful feedback loop. Thus, if we only medicate, whether through alcohol, chocolate, or antidepressants, we might miss out on a whole lot. What might depression be telling me? That I need to move, to change a story I am telling, a belief I am holding, or an activity I am regularly indulging in—or not indulging in. It is telling me that where I am giving my attention, what I am being and doing, does not serve me.

Joy, of course, would be the "keep going" part of this guidance system. If a friendship, job, or situation brings me joy, then I sustain it. I would caution only that we must take time to distinguish between real joy and a fleeting moment of happiness—crack cocaine will, as I understand it, bring you a moment of happiness, but it will not bring you joy. Similarly we might *think* a particular food item will bring us joy. We might have thought this often and come to believe it makes us happy. However, upon closer observation, we might discover this is not the case. Becoming more conscious of what is actually happening when we reach for the chocolate or a glass of wine can be massively revealing. It is possible to access joy, peace, and complete contentment from our own being—no external source is required, even if we are in the habit of believing and practicing otherwise.

When "Bad" Feelings Arise as we Follow our Bliss

Starting to write that book, deciding to create a company, or ending a relationship that no longer serves you—all of these will involve experiences of fear and discomfort. But you can recognize and understand these emotions as being part of the process of creating what your heart truly desires. Indeed, an integral part of this process may be the arising of the very fear that you have always let hold you back. It invites you now to respond differently ... to transcend and transmute it. Every moment is an opportunity to transform and evolve, if we wish.

It's how you feel when you imagine yourself running your own company or receiving an email from the reader who benefitted from your work, or what it would be like to share your life with someone who loves you unconditionally, as you are, which is the truest guide. If you feel joy when imagining a particular dream, this is a clue to explore in this direction.

Clearly a greater familiarity with feelings and distinctions between them is necessary as we look to live life in this way, just as we developed distinctions between healthy and rotten odors when we learned to use smell as a helpful tool. Here is a favorite Rumi poem that reminds us to allow whatever arises, to choose our response. It reminds us that it's all opportunity.

The Guest House

This being human is a guest house.
Every morning a new arrival.
A joy, a depression, a meanness,
some momentary awareness comes
as an unexpected visitor.
Welcome and entertain them all!
Even if they're a crowd of sorrows,
who violently sweep your house
empty of its furniture,
still, treat each guest honorably.
He may be clearing you out
for some new delight.
The dark thought, the shame, the malice,
meet them at the door laughing, and invite them in.
Be grateful for whoever comes,
because each has been sent
as a guide from beyond.
—Jelaluddin Rumi

Exercises

Grab a pen and paper for these chapter-ending
exercises. It will be more effective and will lead
to a deeper process as you write down your
thoughts and reflections.

• Choose a challenge in your life, recent or current.

What's your level of engagement—drama, situation, choice, or opportunity? Is an upgrade possible? What might be the benefits of such an upgrade?

- *Practice responding to life events—maybe beginning with bad driving, your own mistakes, or difficulty in a relationship—with the question "What if I created this?" or "What's the opportunity, the hidden gift, here?" If you want to find an opportunity or gift, it will present itself. You might find resistance to the very possibility; if so, ask "What's the opportunity here?"!*

- *What makes your heart sing? What activities leave you feeling vital, alive, and inspired? How can you wiggle around a bit and feel more comfortable? Set up a plan to do more of these activities in the coming weeks. Commit time to your own well-being and ask others to help you in this commitment as necessary—maybe you can ask them to do the same for themselves.*

Man's perceptions are not bounded by organs of perception; he perceives far more than sense
(tho' ever so acute) can discover.

—*William Blake*

Chapter 9:

Access Your Inner Guidance System (Thinking Optional)

We delude ourselves by believing that what we sense and think describes how it is. In a fundamental sense, we delude ourselves in experiencing this illusory world of form to be objectively real. In fact, we see a projection of our mind. In believing the immeasurable and immaterial to be unreal, we have created an engagement with life that does not work—because such beliefs are incorrect. Simple reason and logic inform us that we need more than reason and logic to navigate life. The evidence of our collective creations—a world that is profoundly dysfunctional by any measure we might apply in assessing another species—screams for a more whole interaction. Our hearts have long been whispering that what the planet cries for now is a new way of being human.

In Chapter 7 of Part One, we looked at one root cause: our belief that we are the ego. Chapter 4 gave examples of how life offers guidance through symbols and synchronicities. Intuition, along with research and reasoning, created clarity in knowing how to respond to being diagnosed without fret or fear. These are not special favors. This guidance and wisdom is accessible to all of us, in every moment. In realizing that life loves us and is supportive of our growth, we open ourselves up to a life of being loved and supported (just as we opened ourselves to a difference experience when we decided that life was meaningless, or a painful endurance test, or merely a means by which to accumulate money and possessions in competition with others). This chapter is designed to help you open to this guidance and inspire you to share your unique gifts more fully as you define and live your life's purpose.

I am a fan of thinking. I enjoy contemplating the implications of the latest neuroscientific research, the connecting pattern in all my intimate relationships, whether Zen Buddhism, *A Course in Miracles*, Advaita Vedanta, the Law of Attraction, and my experience can truly be reconciled, or what to choose from the dinner menu. As awesome as the complete cessation of thought is, I have no desire to reside there the whole time. I also love offshoots of thinking, those great gifts of our culture—reason, logic, and rational analysis. However, it has become clear that thinking is just one lens through which we can engage with the world, just one source of information and understanding. And in believing it is the only or primary one, we expose the limitations of such a means of engaging with life.

Taking time to look at our mind we come to notice how much thinking is not even necessary. We encounter a habitual tangle of past-obsessed and future-fearing waste of time. Lacking any purposeful function, we may also observe a dysfunctional quality which creates much suffering. In learning to allow the mind to quieten through sitting meditation, movement meditation (tai chi, yoga, dancing, etc.), or I don't even know I am meditating meditation, such as leisurely walks in nature, we notice the joy in simply being. We discover that the peace and happiness we were trying to think our way to was here all along. In addition, a quieter mind allows more space for a greater intelligence to be noticed and utilized. This intelligence is experienced as intuition or feeling, of the heart more than the head, and if we are not in touch with it we are utilizing only a fraction of our available intelligence. Which is not very smart—think about it! In living from our heart, we experience a fuller expression of our humanity and develop latent capacities for wiser living.

A belief in thinking as the primary means of arriving at truth, being literally "head-strong," leaves us rather like airplanes without radar. No wonder we are crashing so spectacularly! Let's look at some ways we might switch our guidance systems back on.

First Some Science

In order to begin grasping the bigger picture, we must be willing to put down, just for a moment, our reasoning mind, fire up our right brain (where we access creativity and interpret patterns and symbols), and quieten our left brain (where a lateral and logical approach using language rules). The aim is to integrate the two more fully, for in learning to drop out of our head and into our heart we access our full intelligence and our full humanity.

Not convinced enough to trust your feelings on the matter? Let's look at the scientific evidence. The findings of Neurocardiology—a study of the interaction between heart and brain—helps us discover that there is much more to our intelligence than thinking alone.

Here are three discoveries to support our accessing our inner guidance.

1. The heart along with your gut, has neurons that make up a "little brain." Your heart is physically equipped to be intelligent.

2. Whilst in modernity we have thought the thinking brain to be the residence of greatest human intelligence, research shows that more information travels from our heart to our brain than from our brain to our heart. What does this suggest?

3. As measured by an electrocardiogram (ECG), the electromagnetic field from your heart is sixty times more powerful than the one from your brain. The magnetic component of the heart's field is *5,000 times* more powerful than the brain's, and is measurable three meters away from your body. It can be fun to visualize this field of energy, imbuing it with qualities we would wish to share as we interact.

This suggests we can utilize a far greater intelligence than via thought alone. Could this electromagnetic field be the mechanism by which we sense that some people are best avoided and others worth gravitating towards? Is this the how sometimes we "just know"? A good starting point for a deeper inquiry and practical applications is *The HeartMath Solution*.

Now the mind has opened, we can enjoy some heart-opening exercises—designed to access a greater proportion of our intelligence.

Exercises

> As with all these exercises, if you notice a compulsion to do them all and do them well, acknowledge the advantage of such an approach yet remain open to being guided to doing only those that best serve you right now. Allow the act of doing these exercises to be, itself, a process in learning to trust your intuition, and distinguish it from thinking. A clue—intuition is quieter, has no need to be right, and presents its conclusions instantaneously.

• *Find a comfortable position and bring your awareness to the center of your chest. Breathe in and out, feeling the breath coming in and out through your heart center. Take a few deep breaths and then breathe with roughly equal lengths of in and out breaths as you continue to imagine* this breathing in and out of your heart. If you are strongly visual, you may choose to see white light or another image accompanying the breath. Placing a finger or two on your heart center may also deepen the experience. Continue for three to five minutes. What has changed? What feels different?

This exercise will enhance all other exercises in this chapter. Regular practice will also enhance your mental and physical well-being. Just five to ten minutes a day can greatly enhance quality of life. If this resonates, try for four weeks and notice what shifts.

When you have a question or decision to make and your mind is simply offering reasons for many different options, causing confusion or a sense of being overwhelmed, repeat this breathing exercise. With practice, you can do this anywhere at any time. Initially you may want to step away from other people and excessive noise; however, as you become familiar with the sensations around your heart, you will be able to "drop into your heart" in an instant, with just a breath or two. Let go of thinking and confusion, confess you don't know, and seek guidance from an expanded intelligence. Continuing breathing into the heart, ask the question in clear terms. What you will likely discover is a "knowing." Like with any new skill, mastery will take practice, and, using a radar/radio analogy, you may need to adjust the frequency and repeat the question. However, the knowing is always available. It is experienced as an instantaneous answer that is beyond and above reason. No thinking or argument will precede it. You think the question into the silence of your heart, and from this silence an answer emerges.

You are likely using this capacity in some way already, in "going with your gut," "following your intuition," and so on. Using conscious attention we train this capacity and more reliably discover our "heart's desires" are those which serve our highest good.

• Practice being aware of the field of energy you are emitting wherever you go. This field interacts with the fields of others, and your emotions affect its quality. Play with feeling love and notice the effect it has on others. You may witness bringing others into greater ease and well-being. Could this be helpful in everyday life? As an act of love and in terms of your efficacy as a communicator? It may even help you secure a raise or get a date! (May you use your newfound powers for good!)

• Observe patterns, symbols, and synchronicities that guide your life. Noticing and appreciating this guidance will see it show up more often.

You can search throughout the whole universe for someone more deserving of your love and affection than you are yourself, and that person is not to be found anywhere.

—The Buddha

We need to learn to love ourselves first, in all our glory and our imperfections. If we cannot love ourselves, we cannot fully open to our ability to love others or our ability to create. Evolution and all hopes for a better world rest in the fearlessness and open-hearted vision of people who embrace life.

—John Lennon

Chapter 10:
Fall in Love with Yourself

If I could give you one experience, it would be the experience of being loved—not loved by anyone or because of anything, but *because you are*. Whilst we hope others will give us this, this can only occur when we have learnt to give it to ourselves; when we have brought loving attention to *every* bit of our experience and aspect of our self.

As we grow up we tend to pick up beliefs about needing to do or not do, be or not be in order to be loved. When this conditioning falls away, we are left with a stunning realization: we are loved. We are always loved—utterly independent of anything we do or say or choose. Each breath—our breathing happening—might remind us of this. As we release the collective clutter from our minds this love is free to flow through us and out into the world. Loving yourself is a prerequisite for being of truly useful service in this world. It is at once the greatest gift we can give ourselves and an act of altruism.

As I have traveled around the world visiting spiritual groups, attending countless personal development and healing seminars, connecting with those seeking to bring about social justice or environmental care, and simply chatting with people in everyday life, I have noticed a curious malady that unites us. It is both a symptom and the cause of the very separate self-experience we have come to assume is true. This malady obstructs our full humanity from being fully expressed.

This malady is self-hate or self-loathing. This is unconsciously projected out on to the world and indeed will affect the very circumstances of our life including our physical health. It is an absence of love for ourselves which keeps us from being able to receive the love that is all around us, from friends and family, from the very fabric of existence. We beat ourselves up; label ourselves "wrong." We harm ourselves, often physically. There are plentiful measures of this crisis of the soul or mind in our culture. Physical self-harm, depression, peaking suicide rates, and the like attest to this monster in our midst. It is the elephant in the room, kept well hidden by the fear of being vulnerable and judged by others were we to share. I have, time and time again, witnessed twenty or thirty people in a room *all* nod their heads in compassionate agreement and recognition when one is brave enough to share the experience of their own occasional self-hatred. *Can you relate to this experience? Even if this is not current in your experience, has it been before? Are there aspects of your being that you still judge? Can you give kindness and a warm embrace to this part of your humanity?*

If we buy into the culture of competition, where being the richest, most beautiful, most popular, or "successful" are glorified we will feel insufficient. There will always be someone who seems to have or be more. And as long as we feel we are not enough, we will always seek more by acquiring and conquering. And when we get to where we wanted, we feel we are empty there too. Abundance is not measured by riches— abundance is a feeling of "being enough." When we consistently generate the feeling of abundance, the outer world naturally aligns. Abundance, like happiness and personal or planetary healing, is an inside job.

This business of judging is passed on from one generation to the next. The cultural undercurrent that arises from the blasphemous idea of a god that is apart from us and anything but love is also a root cause of our disconnection. We have believed the profoundly ignorant stories from people who have, because of their own fear and judgment, claimed to know what is real. No wonder we find strident atheism in response to such poor caricatures of infinite intelligence.

There is wisdom in rejecting these old stories.

And we must reject the story that we are mechanisms—mere biological beings— living in a purposeless world of matter, scarcity, and competition, victims of genes and heredity, *adrift in a world of no greater intelligence than that of which we are aware*. For we live by our stories. We can replace these old stories not by bemoaning the darkness, not by judging the world as we once judged ourselves, but by creating a new story, a new worldview, and embodying it—a story that is so luminescent, so evidently less partial, speaking to all levels of our being, that our old, cynical, doubting eyes are blinded by the light.

This loving oneself is not only about our well-being. It is not merely a psychological issue; it is a social, political, and perhaps even survival issue. We are realizing that anything prevalent in our inner worlds is of collective and planetary concern. If I cannot love myself, my capacity to demonstrate concern for you or for the air we breathe is diminished. If I see myself as really worthless, then what spare worth will I have to give you or the world that nourishes us?

You will probably have experienced how your own emotional mood or your own self-view colors your view of another, indeed of life itself. It is easy to see at such times how our view of the world begins with our view of our *self*. Is it mere coincidence that, at a time when the dominant culture on our planet is in the grips of self-loathing, we are destroying that which nourishes us and sustains us? In truth, we are destroying ourselves!

There is a common misconception that we must deny ourselves and give to others first in order to be "good." In truth, to give anything to anyone, I must first possess it. I can offer you only the love present in my experience. If there is a part of me that I loathe, I will loathe it in you. It is only once I have made peace with my foibles and imperfections, my darkness and my shameful secrets, that I meet you, with yours, in peace. It is only when I realize I am whole and complete, *as I am*, that I can see you the same way. My offering you unconditional love is dependent on me first allowing it for myself. Your receiving it is dependent on your relationship with yourself.

We might be wary of such talk of self-love because we are aware of the ugliness of the narcissist, the self that is obsessed with itself. Look closer at such a being and you might see that this posture is merely protection from a magnitude of insecurity and self-loathing—so much that an entire anti-personality was required to obscure it from the conscious mind. We are rightly wary of this form of self-regard as it comes from a wounded separate self. The self-love I speak of comes from (and is an expression of) the integrated being realizing itself as *one* with all things. It is not a narcissistic "I am great!" or "I am better than everyone." It is more like "I am inherently worthy, and I see others as equally so. The world loves me every day, nourishing me with breath and being; who am I to disagree?"

Another common misperception in "spiritual" circles is that one must deny oneself in order to be spiritual or good—or that, as we are ultimately impersonal, we must ignore the personal. Here we find partial understanding arising perhaps when we are unwilling to look at our own darkness. From the vast expanse of the impersonal, there is only love. No edicts or proclamations. Another "spiritual" idea, that of the ascetic, can be an expression of self-judgment, resting on a belief in a god (or goddess) who desires you to suffer to receive their love.

In its wiser form, ascetism or mere self-restraint expresses the *greatest* self-love: we decide we deserve nothing less than the perpetual blissful union with God/Life (and within this union we desire nothing but the Beloved and would not desire anything that would obstruct this). There is no self-denial here unless one has touched only the pleasure derived from a cookie, and imagines it comparable to *being* peace and love. Indeed I would suggest that even your love of Spirit/ Life is proportional to your love of self. To be spiritual is to love for love is Reality's essence. In loving the self, loving others, and loving the world, we realize it's all ultimately the same. It's all, literally, *one*.

Between the extremes of narcissism and self-sacrifice there is a happy middle ground. It is the realization that we are, in our entirety—with our fears and doubts, our judgment, our failures, our petty selfishness, our shallow desires, and harmful actions—lovable. There is perhaps no more precious moment in a human life than when finally we realize—perhaps for the first time—that we are loved and lovable, independent of action. We are loved by virtue of our being. As we love the infant who vomits down our back, pees in our face, and throws food on the floor for the fifth time in one meal, life loves us! For we too know not what we do. Would you treat a child as you treat yourself? Will you commit to giving yourself the same care and love as you would a child?

When we realize our inherent lovability, we can begin to share this unconditional love with the world.

My own journey has included going into dark corners of self-loathing. I have been to a place where I decided

184

that I was worthless. It was only when I cleared the last remaining fragment of this idea—the last piece of shrapnel from a hate bomb I had self-detonated long ago—that this book began to flow.

The reward for this work of learning to self-love is the experience of love itself. From this stems all manner of wonderful consequences. When we are in anything other than loving acceptance, we expend a huge amount of energy on wasteful mind activity. We preen, posture, and prattle on to look cool and be popular. Of course, we only *try* to be cool and popular when we feel uncool or perceive ourselves as unpopular.

To be cool is often to be nothing more than a master of masks and mirrors. We mistakenly seek external salve for an internal wound that ultimately can only be healed from the inside, by our love for ourselves. The energy we once wasted on trying to be someone else is now free to be put towards creative pursuits, starting that business, going on that trip, commencing that community project, and building a new world through our transformed being. Coming from a place of wholeness, a place of love, these creative offerings and this new world will be whole and loving. From this view, we see that the world depends on our falling in love with ourselves … on our allowing unity where there once was division.

The purpose of this chapter is simply to invite an unflinching, loving look at oneself, to ask to what extent do I love myself and how might I make this love more complete? How might I improve my relationship with myself and thus improve all other relationships? Please be mindful not to beat yourself up if you notice yourself beating yourself up! Break the vicious cycle with love.

There are side-effects to developing self-love. As you allow the love that is always here into your experience, you alter the very matrix of energy that is your life. Likely shifts will be that you experience more love and less judgment from others, relationships will grow (maybe that relationship you have always wanted will present itself), and financial circumstances will improve. All that was stopping you before was the confusion that you needed love and abundance from *out there*. In choosing to allow these feelings within yourself, the outer is taken care of, and inner and outer are ever more clearly seen to be *unified*.

Exercises

You may wish to do these exercises alone and with tissues at hand. Be kind and gentle with yourself.

- *Ask yourself: Do I love myself unconditionally? There is no other type of love. If I love myself only when I am cheerful and upbeat or when I am performing well at work or when I am helping others, I do not wholly love myself. We are aiming high here for wholeness, not partiality ... for a solution, not a Band-Aid. This begins with knowing that such full resolution is possible, and first being honest about where you are currently. What parts of yourself do you not allow love? When and during which activities or circumstance do you not love yourself? These are the times of great opportunity where we are invited to offer love in the future.*

- *Write a list of ten desirable qualities you possess. If you have a hard time finding ten, ask your friends to help. Perhaps let them know about this process and invite them to join in. Who, truly, beyond the veneer of cynicism and "I'm fine" could not benefit from more love in their life? See what qualities you bring into the world, what is beautiful in you, and sit with it a while. Realize you are loved as you are.*

- *Write a list of ten undesirable aspects about your behavior or how you perceive yourself. You will likely have less trouble here, but friends may still be able to help if necessary! What you find troubling in someone else will likely be aspects of yourself that you dislike and have thus disowned and project onto others. Include them on this list. Forgive yourself for all of it. Love yourself with it all in mind. Go through each one, stating, for example, "I am impatient, and I love and accept myself. I am arrogant, and I love and accept myself." This may be challenging at first (if it is, make sure you have included "I am self-loathing,* *and I love and accept myself"). Notice what shifts and breakthroughs you experience ... how you now feel. If you feel sad—you guessed it, add "I am sad, and I love and accept myself." This exercise can be part of a process of transformation which begins with making a decision **now!***

- *Consider how you speak to yourself when you have made a mistake. Or the question might be more obvious—how do you speak to yourself generally? Is the tone kind and forgiving? Would you want to speak to anyone else as you dialogue with yourself? If necessary, commit to communicating with yourself more kindly. It might help to consider yourself a manager overseeing an angry or inexperienced staff member, gently and patiently coaching him or her towards a more fruitful and wholesome way of communicating.*

- *Make time each day to appreciate yourself. This might be a five-minute start-of-the-day appreciation for who you are, complemented by a five-minute end-of-day acknowledgment of all the kindnesses and intelligences you displayed throughout the day. We behave as we think we are. Set aside an hour or so—or, even better, a half-day or full day—per week for a month and commit to nourishing your journey towards becoming your ever-more-perfect self. Get a massage, watch an inspiring film, take time to walk in nature, laugh with friends.*

- *Practice daily the following five-minute meditation. You might find you enjoy it so much you want to do it more. Regular practice is the key. Find a comfortable position and bring your awareness to the center of your chest. Breathe in love. On the out breath, feel gratitude for being loved.*

Persist with this practice. It takes a while to perfect self-loathing; it will take a while to replace it with unconditional self-love and acceptance—but the effort will be life changing!

Our deepest fear is not that we are inadequate. Our deepest fear is that we are powerful beyond measure. It is our light, not our darkness that most frightens us. We ask ourselves, 'Who am I to be brilliant, gorgeous, talented, fabulous?' Actually, who are you not to be? You are a child of God. Your playing small does not serve the world. There is nothing enlightened about shrinking so that other people won't feel insecure around you. We are all meant to shine, as children do. We were born to make manifest the glory of God that is within us. It's not just in some of us; it's in everyone. And as we let our own light shine, we unconsciously give other people permission to do the same. As we are liberated from our own fear, our presence automatically liberates others.

—Marianne Williamson

Chapter 11:
Surrender Disempowerment

You may be accustomed to "playing small" as I have been. Victim consciousness is a subtle and powerful conditioner. The fearful and separate self-experience (ego) desperately tries to make itself feel powerful by telling others what to do or what they should be. Thus we are exposed to politicians, advertisements, religious leaders, even teachers and parents who give us inherently disempowering messages that endeavor to stimulate such fear within us that we feel compelled to vote for the party, buy the deodorant, believe in their god, give to their church, or live the life they wished they had lived. Our choice is whether we relinquish our power to others, or choose to express the unique being we are. Even the power of choice is denied us if we choose to believe both neuroscience and some contemporary spiritual teachings that tell us there is no such thing as free will. As ever, if we look more closely, we find here great truth, and partiality.

Is Will Free?

The question of whether the human being is volitional—can actually choose—is a question that has vexed philosophers and scientists for millennia, and with good reason. It is fundamental to how we live our lives and to what degree we are responsible for our life choices. I will attempt here, in a few hundred words, to summarize the debate as I have come to understand it, for statements that we have no free will can be misleading. There is a need to increase the number of empowered beings in our world yet such a statement can cause disempowerment. Our emotional mastery and freedom from suffering depend on this experience of empowerment and personal responsibility. As is often the case, the truth is more complex than such dualistic statements allow.

Benjamin Libet's neuroscience experiments of the 1970s revealed a counterintuitive understanding of brain function: when subjects chose to perform an action, the part of the brain associated with the conscious *me*—the chooser, we assume—was activated *after* the part of the brain responsible for taking an action. One might conclude from this that free will does not exist, yet Libet himself did not assert this. The philosopher Daniel Dennett, suggests there is still room for free will *and* a deterministic universe as mapped out by a mechanistic worldview.

There is another avenue of enquiry through which we can come to question the existence of free will. Just as we can objectively question, we can do so subjectively by analyzing our own experience and realizing the unitive nature of consciousness; here, the usual experience of being a separate independent being dissolves. We experience "just this.". It becomes obvious that I am indeed that. Once again, if that which we have assumed to be the agent of free will—the thinking mind, the separate self—does not exist as we thought, we might reasonably conclude that free will does not exist. In this way much spiritual bypassing (the use of spiritual ideas to avoid the realities of life experience) can occur. In the face of its own suffering and the considerable challenge/opportunity we face, the idea of not having any free will is a most attractive notion for the ego, just as having complete control of life is. I draw attention to this in the hope that we may become more empowered and allow our conclusions on the nature of self to be as nuanced and as helpful as possible.

I know from my own experience that, when I have believed there is no free will, I have acted accordingly and created more suffering for myself and others. When I believe in my capacity to create and effect change, I am able to make choices that really do make a difference. So I merely caution you: choose carefully whether you believe in free will or not. I offer the following simple guide.

Let us assume there are two possibilities and we cannot know which one is true. Scenario number 1:

there is no free will. Scenario number 2: there is free will.

Within scenario number 1, my ability to choose is an illusion; it is, in fact, just a consequence of endless causation, resulting in current subconscious tendencies and brain activity. Therefore, what I choose to believe does not matter. Therefore no choice is preferable over another—it does not matter whether I believe in free will or not. Within scenario number 2, free will does exist, and thus the choice I make is a fundamental determinant in how I experience my life and the extent to which I can show up as an agent of change—or not. I can choose to exercise free will or I can choose not to

Thus, simple logic guides us that, when faced with this uncertainty, we must choose to believe in free will! We otherwise abdicate becoming a glorious agent of change, unable to harness the soul power Gandhi spoke of, but instead playing the victim. This is merely megalomania inverted.

A more nuanced view of what free will might be can be found in regarding it as an emergent property of consciousness. You can have free will, or not, depending on the degree to which you are aware of conditioning and subconscious and emotional triggers. Free will is present to the degree you have transcended your egoic self, or thinking mind, which neuroscience and some spiritual teachings identify as being of limited volitional capacity.

Realizing that we are neither our egoic self nor our thinking mind, we come to understand free will as a capacity we develop, as we develop our consciousness.

Its ultimate expression is reached when we choose to give up our illusory personal autonomy in service to Life or God and, in so doing, we discover that this was always Life/God's will. In other words, my will was merely an expression of Life/God's will. We see, with a very large smile, there is only the will of life itself, giving an aspect of itself the experience of separation, with its own apparently free will, as part of its experiencing itself as individuate and separate ... only then can the experience of union arise. In other words, free will absolutely does and absolutely does not exist! Whilst we are in time and space, in this world, we would do well to believe we have free will—and it is powerful in proportion to our alignment with the whole from which it flows. More delicious paradox!

Again, to draw this back into relevancy within our world, we are agents of change, and we are being invited to step more fully into our power to bring a new world into being. If we choose.

Let us heed the clear communication from masters such as Jesus: "You will do the same works I have done, and even greater works" (John 14:12, New Living Translation), or "The kingdom of God is within you" (Luke 17:21, King James Version). And here are the Buddha's last words, as recorded in the *Mahaparinibbana Sutta*: "Be lamps unto yourselves. Rely on yourselves." Let us realize deeply that it is the wisdom within us that is the most reliable guide. And let us remember that enlightenment, awakening, freedom from suffering, and the like are reasonable goals for any man or woman with a bit of imagination and some resolve. You can experience these things.

Could it be it is time for us to drop our small self-identification and realize the infinite being of great power and unlimited potential we truly are? What's stopping us?

That brilliant integrator of inner transformation and social change, Mahatma Gandhi suggested, "Our greatness lies not so much in being able to remake the world—that is the myth of the atomic age—as in being able to remake ourselves." I would suggest that, from within Oneness, the two apparently separate pursuits are the same, as Gandhi himself knew, and in remaking ourselves we remake the world.

If you want a more loving and just world, remove all that is unloving or unjust within your mind. And perhaps then begin efforts to remake the world; from such an integrated consciousness you might actually be part of the solution rather than perpetuating the problem in different form. Gandhi's wife, Kasturba, was once asked what made her husband so much more effective than other men. She responded that, whereas most of us have conflicting values, feelings, words, and actions, her husband created a unity of words, thoughts, feelings, and deeds. It is in creating such inner unity that free will is at once both most fruitfully exercised and immeasurably enhanced, for all energy can be focused through this prism of inner peace. Such inner harmony is of immeasurable value in a world at war with itself.

I suggest that, rather than disable our free will, the purpose of awakening to our impersonal true nature is to activate our will more powerfully by aligning it with that impersonal vastness, with the intelligence of life itself. In seeing the illusory nature of the ego, discovering ultimately that it does not exist, we are able to allow our desires to be simply expressions of Life's own wishes. We become an agent of Oneness, and our lives are empowered in proportion to the degree we surrender our personality to the impersonal and become of service to the Whole.

Would this not be the obvious evolutionary step in a world in which we have created the possibility of the extinction of our species? We have done this, after all, by believing the story of our being hyper-individuated separate selves, competing in a world of lack and scarcity where only the fittest survive. The new story that is emerging from an awakened consciousness is one in which our essential Oneness is realized, and the scattered efforts of *me* to look after *me* and my own becomes *we* working together to create a more functional world. In this correcting of our course, paradoxically, individual empowerment is key. Thus we are each called to the task—to create love and peace in our being, to be at one in our inner world, not merely for our own contentment, but so this peace may spread to our families, our communities, and to our world.

Joy, peace, love ... they are contagious! Let us become sick with love that we may heal the lesser frequency of fear.

Along with Gandhi, we can look to other figures in history to see what an awakened consciousness is capable of creating. Observing we are endowed with much the same faculties and capacities, we realize how powerful we are.

This world is not an illusion in the sense it does not exist; rather it is an illusion in that it is not as it appears. There are spiritual teachers who say all we see is just *maya*, a Sanskrit word commonly translated to mean "illusion." Therefore, these teachers say, there is nothing to do but watch our karma unfold. There is absolute truth in such statements yet they can be used by the ego for spiritual bypassing. So long as we experience the world, we are called to act within it, whilst remembering, it's just a dream; may our co-creative endeavors be suitably playful.

Be Your Own Master

Consult your own wisdom that you may make your own informed choice. You may wish to apply author Tim Freke's lighthearted rule when assessing spiritual teachings: "Would I give this same advice to my children?"

It seems unlikely that the 14 billion years of life's evolution we hypothesize, which has led progressively to the extraordinary accomplishment of the experience of an individuated personal consciousness, *really* should culminate in the realization that I am nothing and there is nothing to do. This is a profound truth and a startling personal *realization*. It is also a dangerous *belief* to prevail in our world. Much confusion arises when we try to conceptualize mystical insight after hearing or reading a description, because mystical insight can only be *experienced*. In this process of conceptualization, ideas about mystical insight are filtered through an entirely different level of consciousness, and the meaning is completely skewed. For example, in awakening it is seen clearly that ultimately nothing really matters in the way the ego believes. Yet it is entirely foreign for an egoically identified consciousness to believe nothing matters. There are perhaps some truths that are best not spoken about at all. Yet, Truth's ineffability compels us to speak of it.

Ultimately, awakening is a call to action and the arising of a profoundly enlarged care and compassion for all life. Twentieth-century Indian philosopher Sri Nisargadatta Maharaj surmised this paradoxical state of affairs succinctly: "Wisdom tells me I am nothing. Love tells me I am everything. Between the two my life flows."

May our awakened consciousness express the balance of these poles. In surrendering the position of a separate me, each of us is empowered to serve the whole, by the whole, as an integral expression of we. In this unity, I realize that my will and Life's will are one. In this way, free will clearly exists. It's just not mine!

Our humanity is crying out right now, not for victims or megalomaniacs, for this combination has seen us arrive at where we are, but for powerful human beings aware of our Oneness, surrendered to this Oneness, and expressing the wishes of this Oneness through our choices, our being, our whole lives.

It's My Pity Party and I'll Cry if I Want To

It's wise to be aware of threads of victim consciousness lurking in our psyche. Resistance to some of the ideas in these pages might be a red flag. Bringing awareness to such parts of our psyche is part of a new empowered being emerging. Part of a life journey might be to plunge fully into disempowerment and darkness in order to know more of empowerment and light.

Even on a path of self-mastery and empowerment we may subtly continue to give up our power. The poor-me voice is a potential which may be triggered at any time. In becoming aware of this ego activity we can learn to remain as the presence we are; it is not necessary to identify. As we aim for the perfection of being entirely free of identification, we remain aware that we are human and will often fall short. This is not failure; it is a learning opportunity and a chance to practice forgiveness ... to receive the love, to be love. Whether the poor me appears in another or we see it in ourselves, love is the most appropriate response. In seeing the inherent perfection in the apparent other or our self, every such circumstance becomes an opportunity to create a more loving and true world. May we realize the power bestowed in each of us and create a more beautiful world, in our own being, moment to moment.

Exercises

- *In what areas of your life are you accustomed to feeling powerless and playing the victim? How can you choose to behave differently in future? This may involve choosing to change a habit. It might involve speaking your truth in a relationship or exploring being less a victim to emotional states. If you notice there are situations in which you abdicate power, resolve to enhance your free will—humble and surrendered—as a powerful, co-creative being.*

- *To what extent is your life in service of Life? How would it look if it were more so, and how would you feel about this change? Would you gain by giving more?*

- *Choose a day to practice kindness all day. Make kindness your focus above all other choices. Choose simply to be especially kind and helpful. Listen, and be on the lookout for opportunities to serve others. Choose to see every encounter as an opportunity to love. Notice how this changes your experience.*

The fear of death follows from the fear of life.
A man who lives fully is prepared to die any time.

—Mark Twain

Chapter 12:
Prepare for Death and Live Fully

I would suggest that fear of life derives from a fear of death, and thus in becoming prepared to die at any time, we live fully.

Even if you and your loved ones were to somehow escape all grief, separation, and serious illness, you and they will nonetheless die. We have a lifetime to prepare for such an inevitability, yet we typically neglect this task. Consequently, death is commonly an event full of fear, anguish, and suffering, which minimizes opportunities for reflection, reconciliation, and learning. In addition, those around us suffer the more we suffer. Conversely, the better able we are to embrace this reality, others will suffer less.

Facing death becomes an opportunity for all involved. Reports from those who work daily with the dying show that death itself can be experienced with complete serenity, and this diminishes the emotional toll on those around us. Death is seen to be what it is—beautiful and in harmony with life. It is recognized as "life's best invention," to use the words of Steve Jobs.

You might think, "I am more interested in living life now than pondering such imponderables." All the more reason to embrace your mortality, for in being prepared for death we live more fully present, in the now. When I am ready to die in this moment, I am freed from the limitations of the separate self-prison.

Meditation

Don't just do something, sit there.
—Osho

There is no activity (so far as it is one) that I have found more fruitful than meditation. If I could recommend two regular practices to you, it would be to meditate, or at least take some time to be still, to be quiet, and to drink plenty of clean water every day. These have produced the most profound and pronounced results in my life experiments.

Meditation practice allows the control of attention, regulation of emotions, and awareness of thoughts, and in so doing allows self-mastery, the end of suffering, and , through grace, the realization of what we are.

There is now considerable research detailing the benefits of a regular meditation practice. These include multiple positive effects upon our physical and mental health that reach out into all corners of our life. It is becoming a part of the education we give our children.

It is easy to see how new generations growing up with these skills will be better equipped to navigate the demands of life in the twenty-first century.

There are hundreds of different forms of meditation. One definition is being physically still and allowing your mind to do the same. In the beginning, often the first discomforting insight is noticing how busy the mind is! This does not mean we are doing it wrong. It is likely we will pass through many failed attempts before we will be able to sit physically still for prolonged periods without adjusting our posture, scratching our nose, or taking any other unconscious action. Stilling the mind takes most people dedicated, long-term practice.

I experienced considerable benefits during the first months I meditated. I became more relaxed and better able to handle stressful situations. I experienced improved insight into troubling thoughts and feelings and felt generally happier. I also felt more energized and better able to self-manage. Continuing regular meditation practice beyond these early leaps, I have experienced more subtle results; the practice seems more about maintaining newfound well-being than breaking through into new realms of joy. Such leaps do still arise, and I appreciate them as happy side-effects of a consistent practice; however, actively seeking such leaps seems to repel them. In meditation we learn to want what is rather than any special experience or bliss.

Paradoxically, it is a loosening up of wanting something other than the here and now that creates the space for the spontaneous arising of freedom and joy, and through this we are gradually able to be what we are. Bit by bit we are no longer held hostage by our thoughts and feelings. Increasingly we become architects of our intricate inner world and thus of our reality as a whole. In short, meditation can be seen as the foundation for a robust and healthy mind, just as the regular intake of fluids is the foundation for the same balance in the body.

The idea is to approach meditation with no purpose, not even to still our minds. Otherwise we may only be discouraged by the noisiness. Let us sit down and shut up and enjoy allowing the benefits to arise as they do.

It may not be in sitting mediation that we most easily find the stillness and inner quiet, the vast spaciousness from which bubbles joy, creativity, and a sense of connection. A body practice such as yoga or qi gong can be a useful place to start to cultivate meditative awareness. Friends have shared that surfing or dancing are their favored access points to stillness. Chanting and singing can be similarly quietening. Being in nature away from the hubbub of urban life might prepare us for delving into the pristine beauty of our inner world. Engaging in all of the above or using one or two as adjuncts to a daily meditation practice will steadily develop our expanded awareness and give us room to be more conscious, creative beings living life from a broader, deeper and more peaceful perspective.

Learning to be Cool with the Small Stuff

On beginning to meditate, I noticed how highly dysfunctional some of my behaviors were, so I began to retrain my mind to make more fruitful choices. Responding rather than reacting became easier. In responding we live from will and intention rather than from unconscious reactions to shadowy emotions or unexamined thought. Before I began meditating, my response to bad driving would be anger and self-righteousness. My body might convulse; I might shake a fist, offer some curses and maybe a honked horn. And I know now that because of my behavior, harmful stress hormones would flood my body. Curiously the phrase I might yell at others—"You fucking idiot!"—was the very same phrase I would utter at myself in times of hyper-critical self-judgment and self-loathing. I only discovered that I was speaking to myself so very harshly after I had begun meditating and my mind's stream slowed sufficiently for a kinder self-dialogue to occur.

Over time I have developed the attitude of being grateful for such phenomena as bad driving or curious patterns of thought. They can be seen as opportunities to learn, and invitations to know oneself better and develop more fully. I now respond with acceptance and amusement to bad driving. Such instances occur less frequently than when I was driving around as a mass of tense energy, and all of this supports the adage, "What you resist persists." In thinking about this, I have noticed patterns—it seems that precisely the experiences we need in order to grow keep occurring until we learn the lessons they invite. The quicker we see the opportunity in patterns of undesirable occurrences and learn the lesson offered, the quicker they will cease to show up in our experience.

Because I had developed this capacity to meditate and reflect, when the brain tumor diagnosis burst into my life I was able to be cool with that too. I surprised myself with the extent to which I was able to use the experience in support of well-being, growth, and life expansion.

Gratitude

Gratitude is heaven itself.
—*William Blake*

When I first read this idea of Blake's I was perplexed. It seemed an overly bold suggestion. I have since discovered, through experience, that it is true. The state of gratitude is indeed an experience so exalted we might call it heaven.

There is no obligation with the practice of gratitude. It is an invitation to wallow in well-being, and one which, should we accept, brings great joy, especially if we allow it to become our center of gravity.

Such a practice might be useful even for those of us already prone to optimism. Neuropsychologist Rick Hanson offers profound observations about the tendency of the mind to focus more on unpleasant, threatening experiences and less so on pleasurable and fun experiences. Hanson makes the point that, from an evolutionary perspective, this was an intelligent and beneficial adaptation.

Imagine you are attacked by a tiger and somehow escape. It is hugely advantageous for your survival that this experience be seared into your memory, that you remain deeply affected, not just by the sight of a tiger, but by the area in which the attack took place, and even by the sound of rustling in the undergrowth. Retaining this memory could well be the difference between your sudden, violent end, and your survival. It is important to understand what is happening in your brain during times of threat or fear of attack. During such a threatening assault, a powerful series of neuronal nets is created by the traumatic events, and these nets are activated by any hint of a repeat of the original experience. On the other hand, if we eat an amazing mango—each bite a joyous, sensory delight—there is less advantage to our survival in remembering the experience vividly.

Our current human experience is, of course, rather different to that of our forebears, but our peace and happiness can still be interrupted by such previously useful, instinctive stress responses to "danger." We seek joy, and yet our brains remain wired and our minds remain conditioned to fear the "danger." In Hanson's terms, our minds act like Velcro for negative experiences and Teflon for positive experiences. This message offers great hope, for we now know and understand more of the neuroplasticity of our brains. Whilst we might be biased by social or evolutionary conditioning and therefore function in a certain way, we are able to use our minds to rewire our brains—and in turn we can alter our minds in a circle of awesomeness. We are beginning to wake up to our power. Far from being victims of genes, circumstance, or conditioning, we are discovering that we are, in fact, architects of our life experience. The positive change we can bring into our lives is proportional to the extent we explore this, discover it to be true in our own experience, and do the work of letting go of the fearful being we once were.

Gratitude is a consequence of being fully present. In addition, gratitude is a powerfully transformative practice. Here is a selection of exercises focused solely on developing our capacity for appreciation.

1. *Grab a pen and paper and begin writing "I am grateful for …"; then list anything and everything that you appreciate in your experience. It might look something like this: "I am grateful for the joy I feel when I see sunlight sparkling in dewdrops, being able to see, chocolate brownies, my family, the love my family give me, my favorite books, for laughter, for sex, for orgasm, for beauty in all its forms …" Keep going until you have filled in two large notebook sheets at least. You may find that you wish to carry on—it is so much fun! If you find yourself thinking—and believing—that*

you cannot find anything more to be grateful for before you've filled in an entire two pages, notice that, by acknowledging these feelings of "done-ness," you are actually committing to feelings other than gratitude. Be grateful for noticing this resistance and keep going! On completing this exercise you will likely feel grateful for having remembered how utterly awesome life is. The more awesome you perceive your life to be, the more awesome it becomes. A daily gratitude practice is a very powerful transformative tool.

2. *Repeat the above exercise in a beautiful spot in nature, but express your gratitude out loud. Sing it to the sky and keep going for at least half an hour. Discover the fact that, in recognizing such a detailed litany of sources of joy and delight, there is simply no room for the self-pitying self to exist. So dazzling is the accumulative light that joy naturally emerges. We also observe our capacity to create emotions, moods, and perspectives.*

3. *The third practice is to start and/or end every day by writing or reciting at least a few sentences that express what you are grateful for. Whilst the first two exercises in this section are introductory exercises, this is an ongoing practice that will yield much well-being. Make it your habit it for a week and observe the results.*

4. *Take a moment before eating a meal to look at each component, to visualize each ingredient, and begin to feel gratitude for how the meal all*

came together. Perhaps thank the person who made it, whether another or yourself, then feel gratitude for the people that produced each item, the people in the shop who sold it, those involved in transporting the goods, the animals that may have given their lives to nourish your body, the farmers, the nourishing soil, and the sunlight. Within thirty seconds, the web of life that was activated in order for you to eat becomes clear. It is a wonderfully illumining experience to see just how interconnected and dependent upon each other we really are. And the meal tastes better. Of course this is most powerful with organic local produce!

5. *This practice is for advanced practitioners: practice being grateful for everything—even, and especially, the difficult and painful stuff! I call this Radical Gratitude and will explore this more deeply in a future work.*

Cultivate Curiosity

Why am I here? What is reality? What happens when I die? What do I value the most? Does my life reflect my most important values? How do I wish to be remembered? What would I change about my life if discovered I might die in six months? What holds me back from making these changes now? Will I now make them?

It is highly likely that there will come a time in every life when such questions become very important. If it doesn't happen long before death, then it probably will when it becomes apparent that death is near. Finding deeper meaning is a huge task to commence at such a time. By fully answering such questions now, when death is not an imminent threat, and then living according to these answers, we avoid the misery of looking back and seeing our deeper truth when it's too late—the incongruence with life as we lived it. Realize you are dying now, for we are dying from the moment we are born.

The inspirational image of the joyous geriatric undertaking some huge life change is a popular one. I enjoyed the film *Beginners* in which an older man is diagnosed with terminal cancer and is thus inspired to come out as gay to his family. The film captures the joy that naturally arises when we are living authentically—especially when death is known to be close. We can live our lives primarily as economic units. We can play a particular role based on how we think someone else expects us to be. But there will always be that deeper part of us seeking to emerge and express who we really are and claim the experience of joy and contentment that naturally follows that blast of authenticity.

Of course it is best to use your energy and resources now and live in peace and contentment for the years to come rather than just the last days. I would rather a day of the joyful peace that results from an effective ordering of my life than to live another fifty years without it.

Get the Deathbed Stuff Out of the Way Now

How many people die with agony in their hearts from not having expressed love or forgiveness to a particular person? Or from not having expressed gratitude to someone or in general? Or for not having done something? How many people on the brink of death look back and wish they had made their lives fundamentally different? How many look back at a life filled with joy and gratitude?

How different an experience will death be for each of us? Will you face death wishing you had gone to the Bahamas, thanked your parents, kissed a particular person, written a novel, retired ten years earlier, or allowed yourself to experience gratitude?

If there remains anything important to you that you have left undone or not attempted, the pain will come when you realize that your journey is almost done, even if it be for only a split second before your life ends. For at that point, the claim "I don't have the time" or "It's not possible" will, for the *only* time, become absolutely true.

The Story of Your Life

In general the universe seems to me to be nearer to a great thought than to a great machine. It may well be, it seems to me, that each

*individual consciousness ought to be compared to
a brain-cell in a universal mind.*
—Sir James Jeans

*Every decision you make
stems from what you think you are.*
—A Course in Miracles

*Whether you think you can, or you can't,
you're right.*
—Henry T. Ford

*The greatest discovery of my generation
is that a human being can alter his life
by altering his attitudes of mind.*
—William James

I could offer a thousand such quotes from countless wisdom traditions and philosophies from across all ages and places. Basically this premise—what you focus on, you will manifest—is the discovery and teaching of *every* sage, master, and inspired scientist I have encountered. And its truth has been made graphically clear to me in my experience.

We are millennia on from the first expressions of this philosophy, and the power of our minds is a more commonly recognized and talked about idea today, yet how much do we use the information that we are indeed powerful beings. In truth, the idea that our inner and outer worlds are separate, our ideas of time and space, and our experience of being separate from one another and, indeed, all of Nature, are but ideas. Great ideas, useful ideas, ideas which make this beautiful realm what it is, yet ... just ideas. If the universe is all thought, ideas, or consciousness, then our inner world—the thoughts and feelings you are entertaining right now—become of cosmic importance. When we see that, on a deeper level, there is no separation between our inner and outer worlds, it becomes obvious that our lives are reflections of our inner worlds—our thoughts, beliefs, intentions, and feelings. Our own empirical analysis confirms this. *Consider how you have already noticed this symbiosis to be true in your experience.*

We can see how the collective story of our times—that we are competitive animals/machines in a biological race to accumulate things and dominate others, as consumers, in a random and meaningless universe—has led to where we are as a society today. Clearly it's an ineffective story for maximizing the well-being and happiness of most. It also happens to be a very partial and biased reading of the evidence. Happily, I believe we are in the process of taking a broader look and creating a new collective story. From this, a new world is being born.

In my own experience, I have witnessed this inner/outer flow as one. For much of my life, however, I unconsciously bought into the negative story of our times that I've just described. I also added my own garnishes, such as "I am unlucky." Then one day, as described in Chapter 6, I became consciously aware of my "I am unlucky" belief. I began to update this belief to better reflect the facts: that if you live in England and have good health and plenty of food and shelter, it is ignorant to consider oneself unlucky. If, in addition, you have loving parents and a great education, it is a delusion of high order. A funny thing happened when I changed this belief to "I am lucky." I became luckier still! And this new and wonderful belief has fed on itself, becoming a circle of awesomeness (the opposite of a "vicious" circle!). Often people will look at my life—its sheer, apparently serendipitously perfect unfolding, with success, even in spite of stupidity, carelessness, and bad habits—and ask, "How did you get so lucky?" Clearly much good fortune, such as place of birth and so on, plays a part. Ultimately all that we are has been given to us, yet we can become more or less, depending upon our attitude. I might say I am so lucky simply because I have long believed that I am.

How life developed under the belief "I am unlucky" was so startlingly at odds with how it developed under the belief "I am lucky" that I finally began to see how the story I *told* of me and my life *became* the story of my life. This was made even clearer when I explored holding beliefs such as "I am a worthless piece of shit" following an experience in which my actions caused great hurt to someone I cared about deeply. It became clear how the choices I made, the habits I indulged in, the hopelessness I felt, were all consequences of this belief.

I became aware of this self-talk only after I began meditating. I remember clearly the shock of hearing me refer to myself as "a fucking idiot" in response to some minor foolishness. I then became appalled when I realized this voice had been playing in my head for a long time. Having become aware of this destructive negative wiring, I began the task of undoing it and replacing it with a more up-to-date view. And guess what? Installing different inputs again created different outputs through life experience. Overall I came to see very clearly that the more gloriously wonderful my *story* of self and life became, the more gloriously wonderful *life itself* became. This, in turn, creates a still more gloriously wonderful story of self and life, and we have once again created a circle of awesomeness!

To live the life that we seek, to be more than we currently are, we must first *think* and *feel* the life we want. It's simple. This is the law of attraction: like attracts like. Is it easy to change an entire operating system? No, but it is possible. It does require a degree of commitment and personal responsibility most are not willing to engage in. Some people will experiment with such a notion, and having laid down a few positive thoughts atop a mountain of negativity, they will continue to get negative results and conclude that such "stuff" does not work. The law of attraction is thus ridiculed, and these people will carry on living the same lives of quiet despair they have endured for years. If they are lucky, their suffering will escalate sufficiently that they will once more be prompted to look at ways they might change and suffer less. I have experienced this cycle myself.

The journey towards self-mastery is a long one. All the more so if you are, as I have been, stubborn and opinionated, and have created quite a mess (and mass) of disempowering beliefs and states of feeling. I see now how my own process of change created a level of direct experience of transformation, which is unusual and enables me to better serve others in their own journeys. Because I went so low and so far into darkness and ignorance, my now luminescently joyous and abundant life serves as an example of what is possible in terms of transformation. In addition, I have tried and tested perspectives and practices that I can now share and encourage others to implement in order to create similar leaps forward in their own life experiences.

Most teachings about profound change, and indeed even the necessarily pithy nature of the quotes at the beginning of this section, leave us short of recognizing the tools and processes we require to apply this deep truth. In pointing to the simple principle, the quotes fail to mention that this task of transforming our being is, in practice, multi-faceted, complex, and subtle. And, of course, it varies from person to person. It's lucky we have our own inner guidance system.

This book provides information that will give any explorer a good start in such a process; however, ultimately a book can offer only a sketchy map for you to guide your own exploration. I have included minimal transformative processes in this book and opportunity to discover more in the Further Reading section at the back. And as was highlighted in Chapter 7, some form of "shadow work"—a process by which we come to know the part of our being in which we have deposited all that we were unable to experience or willing to allow as part of us—is essential too. A shadow with which we have no familiarity or relationship can sabotage all our efforts to evolve and manifest. A shadow owned and loved allows a unity of being from which great power flows. *The Dark Side of the Light Chasers* by Debbie Ford is a useful introduction to this work. Daily dipping into such books and completion of the exercises in this book catalyzes awakening and transformation. Waking up is at once a moment's insight and one long reminding.

When we seek positive change and make clear we are willing to do the work and take action, unseen effects result. Life will respond with the necessary guidance and "apparent" chance encounters. As I learn ever more deeply, we need not concern ourselves with the details; once we *persistently and consistently* hold a clear intention in our minds and a good feeling in our hearts to accompany it, the vibrational nature of this mystery will take care of the rest.

So, let's be clear on what is necessary, along with being prepared for death, to live your most wonderful and extraordinary life:

1. *Become aware of your stories. The two primary meta-narratives—the driving creative forces in your life—are your "self story" and your "life story." Together, they form your life.*

*Your self story: What have you decided you are?
How do you see yourself? How do you dialogue
with yourself? Who do you think you are? What
have you decided you are and are not capable of?
Do you feel good about yourself? Do you consider
yourself worthy and deserving of love, health, and
wealth? Are you powerful or not?*

*Your life story: Is life meaningful and purposeful?
Is it pointless and cruel? Does life love you or not?
Are there laws and principles that you can use for
the benefit of yourself and those around you? Are
you mostly grateful or resentful for being alive?*

*Of course what is useful here are not simply the
answers you might give with your conscious mind
but the thought patterns and beliefs that a deeper
enquiry and noticing of your inner world will reveal.
We must make a commitment to be deeply honest
with ourselves and answer the questions not
simply as we would like.*

2. *Upgrade your stories. These stories are your
operating software and require ongoing upgrad-
ing as new data and desires come into your
awareness. This may sound a little tedious: a
bit like hard work. It is far less tedious than
experiencing an unconsciously created life
full of negativity. It is far less hard work than
forever cleaning up the messes you have made
by self-sabotaging and limiting perspectives*

221

and beliefs. With practice, this becomes an entirely effortless and enjoyable process. It is worth the effort!

But What if it's Not True?

If you believe it's true that changing your story will change your life, it's true for you, and your experience will reflect that truth. And vice versa. It also works the other way—our experience informs our beliefs. Do you see connections between attitudes, beliefs, and self-images you have held and how your life experience has unfolded?

A key misperception we must dissolve here is that, when we speak of "reality," we are, as an objective and separate self, merely pointing to our perception of what is "out there" and separate from us. The awesome discovery is that *we are never merely defining; we are always creating.* In every moment of our experience we are in symbiotic exchange with this life *that we are.*

The extent to which you believe this to be true determines the extent to which you will experience life this way. This creative aspect to the human experience is in operation regardless of what we think, regardless of whether we insist "stories are just stories"; "I don't care what my story is"; "I have transcended all stories"; "I am not interested in my story"; "I am spiritual"; or "I am a powerful, co-creative being." If we attempt to abdicate and deny or simply be unaware of our co-creative power, we simply create the experience of being powerless.

We must first drop outdated superstitions before we can truly empower our being and step forward into the delightful creative dance we came here to experience. Here are some examples of such superstitions:

- *I am separate from the world.*
- *Thoughts and feelings are immaterial; they are not so important because we live in a material world.*
- *I am just watching.*

These can now be seen as "bugs" in the old operating system. In each moment we are called to let them go and replace them with information that is current to our personal life experiences, and indeed what the latest science actually suggests. As ever, experiment for yourself and discover what is true for you.

It's Absolutely Relative

It is to be hoped that all seekers of truth eventually come to a place in their journey when they realize that there is no one philosophy or belief system that is absolutely or exclusively true. No matter how comforting it might be to believe that my worldview is true, it's partial at best. It's most helpful to look at perspectives, whether of the self or of the world, in terms of their functionality—the effect they have.

All truth on the relative level—that which can be written or spoken of—is partial. This truth likely arises, for many people, alongside a realization of the paradoxical nature of truth itself. We come to see that reality has no problem whatsoever in being both "this" and "that" simultaneously. We can easily see this by noticing how different people or the same person at a different time will view the same circumstance in a different way. Or by realizing that we can be, at once, selfish and generous—or wise and foolish. In any of these cases, the view I feel more deeply becomes more true in my experience. Quantum physics has experimentally confirmed that matter can truly simultaneously be *this and that*: it is not a particle *or* a wave but a particle *and* a wave. Rather than being any one thing, it is in a state of potentiality.

So are you! We come to see in our own lives that, besides existing as the basic level of matter, we are potential: *itself* becoming ever more *itself*. How's that for an enticing and inspiring belief?

More delicious paradox! Paradox is, as English writer G. K. Chesterton pointed out, "Truth standing on her head to get attention." Beyond the apparent contradiction, if we look more deeply, we will see the higher order of unity from which it appears paradoxical, and thus our perspective becomes one of a higher unity.

It is our destiny never to be able to define or know ultimate reality conceptually, and thus we learn that *it becomes a question of choice*. Life is a blank canvas upon which you paint your experience. Learning to do so consciously is mastery. When we realize this, choosing a view that brings joy takes priority. Let's look at an example—a big, juicy one—the existence of God. Many people believe in God, whatever this might mean to them. In response, others feel the need to disbelieve in someone else's idea of God. Others say we cannot know, and still others prefer not to get involved.

In recent years, advances in physics have come up with many remarkable discoveries. One of particular interest here is the discovery of the Zero Point Field. This energy field is present in everything and everyone; it contains all information from all time; our very being depends on our interaction with this energy. It is a void of sorts, yet it is not really empty; in fact, it is that from which all arises—a continuum where reality pops in and out of existence. Sounds a bit like an aspect of a more subtle conception of a divine power, no?

Those with a "spiritual" view of life will find much here to align with ideas of the *Godhead* or *Consciousness*. The books *The Field* by Lynne McTaggart and *The Holographic Universe* by Michael Talbot are fascinating and easy introductions to scientific research that points to life being more a magical mystery than mere mechanistic matter. There are even scientists, such as Amit Goswami, retired professor of theoretical physics and author of *God Is Not Dead*, who cite such scientific discoveries as evidence of the existence of God. Of course here we use the word "God" in a far more subtle way than we find in most religious expressions, or the reactions to them, atheism or agnosticism. Here "God" is more principle or energy field than father-like being.

However, many spiritually minded thinkers will find such a connection troublesome, even if they are unable to refute the simple logic. It comes down to two opposing beliefs or stories of reality, neither of which can ever be proven, although we can have a jolly good argument about it. Whether you call it God or the Zero Point Field is merely a consequence of many prior beliefs and assumptions. Each is as true or false as the other.

Again we are presented with the possibility of accepting that such matters of fundamental truth cannot be given to us by science or a pre-packaged belief system. We cannot know, and we are thus left with the awesome possibility of consciously choosing a worldview. Unencumbered by the notion that we must accept wholesale any particular worldview or tradition as true, we are free to try on what works. Quite naturally, we will work towards adopting perspectives that *yield more joy and less suffering for us and others.*

Exercises

* *Common advice for those facing death is to get their affairs in order. Of course, we are all facing death—are your affairs in order? I don't mean have you written a will or made plans for who will look after your pet; is your experience of joy at a*

level you are content with? Have you done, or are you taking steps to do, all you wish to do? Are you giving/serving/creating as much as you would like? Why not write that book, sign up for those singing lessons, or enquire about the training for a new line of work? Do it now! Is there something you need to say to someone?

- *Look at the five most common regrets of the dying and see which areas might offer potential for you. These were compiled by Bronnie Ware, an Australian nurse who worked in palliative care for several years, caring for people in the last twelve weeks of their lives. If you wish to explore further, she has shared these jewels of wisdom in her book, The Top Five Regrets of the Dying: A Life Transformed by the Dearly Departing:*

  1. I wish I'd had the courage to live a life true to myself, not the life others expected of me.
  2. I wish I hadn't worked so hard.
  3. I wish I'd had the courage to express my feelings.
  4. I wish I had stayed in touch with my friends.
  5. I wish I had let myself be happier.

Let's learn from the mistakes of others. If you were to die now, which of these would you also regret? Pick the one you feel strongest about and take action to improve your experience today to the extent that, if you were to die tomorrow, your regret would be lessened.

• Write out who you are and what life is for you. Make sure the assumptions, beliefs, and perspectives by which you live are explicit in your mind. Ask these questions: Does this serve me? Is it true? Does my life reflect it? Is it the best story I can tell?

Write an improved version and revisit it daily, perhaps writing out a new version each day for a period of time until you see you are living the changes you have installed into your operating system.

You must live in the present, launch yourself on every wave, find your eternity in each moment. Fools stand on their island of opportunities and look toward another land. There is no other land; there is no other life but this.

—Henry David Thoreau

Chapter 13:
This Is It!

This is it. This is the end of all seeking of enlightenment, all searching for God, all wanting to know the truth. And it is the beginning of a new phase of allowing *This*, which has been found to be expressed in each step, in each word, in each breath. And *This* was here all along. It's with you now. It *is* you now. We can call this non-dual consciousness, Buddha nature, being, presence, awareness, awakening, god, or God. *This* is unconcerned with names. We might be wisest to keep silent, for it is in the quiet that *This* is most easily heard. Yet there is a sublime quality to This that one feels obliged to share. It is a secret that begs to be revealed. Unlike the untouched travel destination that becomes crowded and commercialized as more people learn of it and visit, *This* is not diminished the more people know about it and converge upon it. *This* is perfect as it is. If we choose to use any label at all—and our compulsion to speak of *This*, to share *This*, to point at *This* rather requires it—we might only consider whether our words help us remember and realize *This*. I call it *This*, lest I look somewhere other than here or now.

This is beyond all beliefs and ideals; *This* is the direct experience of *This*. *This* is This experiencing itself via the experience of I am—how utterly mysterious and exquisite!

This is the universe, *This* is God, *This* is you, me, and the Milky Way. *This* is everything, seen and unseen. *This* is nothing. It is the words you read, you the reader, and the mysterious process of reading, of understanding, and misunderstanding—all at the same time! How does this communication occur or fail to occur? Who are you? Who am I? How are we at once able to experience ourselves as *This* and also as separate from *This*? If you find yourself perplexed, see your confusion as the communication having in fact occurred, and enjoy *This*. For *This* is right in front our eyes and an unseeable mystery. *This* is all we know and yet it is unknowable.

We are *This*.

If you are laughing, you probably know what I am writing about here, or perhaps you just noticed now. Whilst we consider ourselves to be the character—in my instance, Will Pye, or *me*, this thinking voice, this stream of consciousness—we are at the same time *This*—the ocean, each blade of grass, a dog turd, mountain spring, and your neighbor from down the street. If we look closely at *This*, for ourselves, or perhaps just to see it, we notice there is just *This*, and it includes me. Or, to put it another way, *This* is just me. Except that, upon this realization, *me* disappears. In awakening, orgasm (in French, *la petite mort*, or the little death!), listening to the most sublime music, we can see that *This* ceases being *me*.

If these ideas all sound rather incomprehensible, it is because they are. Reality itself is this *and* that— neither and both at once. To be fair to our language, this finite capacity to describe *This* is more due to the infinite nature of *This* than any mere limitations of language. For language occurs within *This*, and, clearly, the fact that something occurs within something else precludes that very something from encompassing that within which it occurs.

This is perfect. Always. Even your habit of believing it is not perfect—perhaps when pain or something other than your preference appears—is perfect. Realization of this truth is freedom. For when you recognize everything— death, life, poverty, riches, pain or pleasure, being liked or loathed—as sweet expressions of *This*, the idea that it can ever be a problem dissolves.

A taste of *This* is sufficient for you to desire only to be *This*, which is great, because *This* is all there is! Except *This* is infinite, and the ways of knowing it and tasting it are perhaps infinite too. And part of tasting *This* must always include not tasting *This*. As if it were possible! Which it is! This (*This*) is a mystery.

Sometimes *This* is experienced as complete accep- tance, peace and harmony, sublime tranquility, and appreciation. Other times, *This* is experienced as fear or sadness or the desire for a cigarette or a super green smoothie. Sometimes *This* desires nothing, knowing it is all here now, and sometimes *This* desires a fuller expression of *This*, knowing all is expanding and grow- ing. Sometimes *This* desires to die to wanting. Sometimes *This* seeks to come into closer contact with what I truly and most deeply desire. Then *This* laughs when it realizes again that *This* is *It*.

Enlightenment, God, Happiness—*This* is it.

The end of all our exploring will be to arrive where we started and to know the place for the first time.
—*T. S. Eliot*

It's Always Now

There exists only the present instant ...
a Now which always and without end is itself new.
There is no yesterday nor any tomorrow,
but only Now, as it was a thousand years ago
and as it will be a thousand years hence.
—*Meister Eckhart*

Nothing has happened in the past;
it happened in the Now.
Nothing will ever happen in the future;
it will happen in the Now.
—*Eckhart Tolle*

People might sit in meditation for thousands of hours in the hope that they will experience reality directly, unfiltered or fettered by thought, which can only ever happen now. It is one thing to *understand* the power of now—

and a good start—it is another to *realize* it. It is easy to grasp intellectually that everything always happens *now*. It is considerable grace to *experience* that this is all there is. Whether we are seeing there is only this now, conceptualizing there is only the present moment, or thinking of a time in the future when we are doing one or the other, it is all happening now.

Can you relax, be happy (even in the presence of sadness), be at ease now? Cultivating this capacity is the path to freedom. This path starts and ends now. This freedom is now.

The only thing that matters is how you are being now. If you consistently realize this, the future will take care of itself.

It is such a simple concept that the complex and thought-loving mind will spend a lifetime disputing it, rather than letting go of complexity, of obsessing about regrets and hopes.

Now is your enlightenment, now is your freedom, now is always available for your appreciation.

Joy is only ever found here, right now. Quit imagining you will find happiness, joy, fulfilment, or peace anytime other than now. Call off the search; it's all here and now.

> *Here it is—right now.*
> *Start thinking about it and you miss it.*
> *—Huang-Po*

This, Too, Will Pass

Everything is in flux.
—Heraclitus

Of all the world's wonders
which is the most wonderful?
That no man, though he sees others dying all
around him, believes that he himself will die.
—The Mahābhārata

A story is told in which a king asks his wisest men—his advisors, philosophers, priests, and scientists—to come up with one sentence that is true in every circumstance. They go away and ponder for days and come back with "This, too will pass." Consider a stressful circumstance in your life and see if this applies. Does it help to keep in mind that what is happening now will cease to happen? Unhappiness will yield to happiness, frustration will become contentment, problems will be resolved, circumstances will change. Just as the storm passes, the clouds part, spring comes, and wounds heal, our inner experience is forever in flux.

Ultimately this phrase points to one of the Buddha's key teachings, that of impermanence. This can be seen as a jewel of Buddha's teaching, a realization that leads to many others. The cessation of suffering and selflessness all rather naturally follow from a moment-to-moment realization of impermanence. One can understand it as a concept easily—from observation or from scientific understanding one can grasp intellectually that everything is in flux … in motion. We can easily see that it is a trick or illusion of consciousness when we experience an emotion, circumstance, or *this life itself* as anything other than a never-ending process … as perpetual motion. It is most helpful to realize this impermanence … to experience this impermanence.

Remember, this includes you!

You are not standing beside this river of time endlessly morphing. You are part of it, a drop flying from one rapid to the other—or the whole river. You, too, will pass. Funnily enough, when we realize this—the impermanence of ourselves—we realize we are that which is deathless. In dying to self, we are born to eternal life. We realize we are awareness itself.

As we allow this realization to permeate our entire being every moment, we are graced with the realization of its eternal beginning and cessation. This is freedom. This is the end of suffering.

You could die at any minute. Meditate on that. Notice that any fear surrounding this passes, just as you will. Notice that which does not pass. Notice the noticing, for it is always noticing. Perhaps we find that the noticing continues even as our bodies and egos cease.

This whole process is a moment's realization, but requires a lifetime of embodiment. However, this realization, this acceptance of your death, this seeing yourself *as the seeing* can only happen now. If you are carrying on reading without accepting this thought, stop a minute. I guarantee that experiencing the dissolving of the contraction, the idea of me, into this expanse, into this laughing expanse, is far more fun than any words to come.

Take a moment, invite grace to tea, want truth now, take a look at what is looking.

And enjoy whatever unfolds—enlightenment or confusion. If it's a taste of enlightenment, stop reading, look some more, soak it up, let your mind be without stimulation for a while. If it's confusion—awesome! For you can still look forward to the taste to come, and it will.

Remembering that this, too, will pass can be a wonderfully effective way to ease suffering. It is easier to allow difficult or painful emotions to arise when we know they will fall away.

I have found the most direct route to the cessation of suffering is to realize the impermanence of me.

Who are You?

There is nothing in life to which we can cling
without suffering, even our own selves.
—*Jonathan Paul Gross*

Perhaps we might say "*especially* our own selves." For clinging is always at the root—clinging to the idea of the me that wants this, needs that, fears the possibility of, and so on. If we can let go of this fundamental clinging, then all else at least diminishes. Until, perhaps, ten seconds later when the self reinvents itself, maybe as the enlightened one or one who is having this very spiritual experience. And so we let go of that too. Laughter helps at this point.

This ever re-emerging nature of the sense of a personal self, separate and self-contained, is a wonder to watch. Whilst one route to realizing impermanence is to imagine your own dying, it is perhaps easier and more powerful to notice, in this moment, the ever-dying-and-being-reborn self-experience. It's just a construct—a really marvelous and oh-so-convincing construct. When we see this, we cannot suffer, for we are not that which suffers.

This is a very clear and memorable part of the experience of the self—recognizing the ego re-emerging after the bliss of *being This*. How utterly wonderful is this capacity for this oneness to experience itself as this apparently separate being. It's a miracle—literally, a marvelous miracle. Let us allow it, along with any other evidence of *me*—and of course there is plenty! This oneness is even more clear after this awakening experience—it becomes a source of resistance and thus suffering *within the very same self-structure that is believing the thought it should not be.* From the expanse of this presence, ego is simply loved—another phenomenon to delight in.

That the self is an illusion does not mean it does not exist; it merely means that it is not as it seems.

The Buddhist scholar Stephen Batchelor has offered

his own translation of Annata, the Buddhist concept that points to selflessness. It does not mean "no-self," he contends, but "not-self."

Focusing on our impersonal true nature is a wonderful thing. It might require we de-emphasize the personal. However, let us not get stuck in this view, which is problematic in two ways:

1. *It is a view that is arising from the very "selfing" experience it decries. The impersonal does not care about emphasizing the impersonal. Only the personal does.*
2. *It's not all impersonal. Enlightenment itself depends on the experience of being a separate me. Wise adults do not dismiss a chance to be as children and indulge in joy, playfulness, and innocence just because they have passed eighteen. We are this impersonal awareness and the individuated consciousness itself too. I find the most truth and the most capacity to love when I celebrate both.*

Exercises

1. *Smile.*
2. *Breathe.*
3. *Smile some more.*

Tell me, what is it you plan to do with your one wild and precious life?

—Mary Oliver

You don't get to decide how you are going to die.
Or when. You can only decide how you are going to live. Now.

—Joan Baez

Chapter 14:
So, What is Important Now?

This is *the* question of my little adventure. The thing I asked myself upon being diagnosed with a brain tumor and the one I invite you to ask yourself now and every day. When I encountered these words right after my diagnosis, I realized the great importance of diving deep into this question and answering it in the most considered and heartfelt manner possible.

What is important now? I would answer, "Being a source of love and truth in the world." Indeed, I have been saying this for many years. My life is beginning to be a more convincing answer in itself. This process of creating unity of thought and action is ongoing.

What is your answer? What is truly important now for you? And, now the clincher: to what extent does your life currently reflect this answer? Does what you do and who you are align with your answer? Be completely honest. Are there choices, behaviors, activities, and attitudes that are contradictory to your stated greatest importance? You see, I can *say* that being a source of love and truth in the world is most important to me; however, if I then, for example, choose to have a second glass of wine and time online watching pornography, then is what I am *doing and being* coherent with my stated values and desires? I might conclude that I am out of alignment: there is a contradiction between my verbal answer and how I am actually living. Equally, I might reason there's nothing "wrong" with pornography, red wine has health benefits, and I don't believe I will go to hell for masturbating, so why should I not "let off a little steam?" Perhaps because the steam can be better directed elsewhere, to a greater advantage?

I have found that there are ways to justify just about anything; for example, the human capacity to rationalize away even the most obvious hypocrisy and horrific war crimes is evidenced with regularity in the media and by our political leaders. It can be revealing to note the same capacity and tendency to justify negative behavior in my own mind. And, of course, whilst I cannot change the minds of the powers that be, I can change mine. I see this tendency for justification especially clearly with regards to behaviors that, whilst not in themselves harmful to others, do not serve my greatest truth or personal values. And it's also interesting to note that it is important for me to desire to bridge the gap between what I *say* is important, and what my life shows to *be* important. A truly joyous life is built on the realization that there's really only one answer—one relevant and true answer. This is found not in our mere words but in our very lives—how we are using our time, energy, and attention. Or as Elmer Green, pioneer of biofeedback puts it: "If you feel that you know a truth, you must be able to demonstrate it in your life to some degree. Otherwise, you don't really know it, you are only talking." Where in your life are you "only talking" and where would you like to be "fully walking"?

You can say that your family and having fun are the most important aspects of your life, but then you might notice you spend more time at work than with your family or pursuing fun activities. You can say that being healthy and happy are most important; however, do you consistently demonstrate the necessary kindness to yourself and your body for this to really happen? Are you happy when you make the occasional "unhealthy" choice?

Is there another option, a better way for you and those you love? To what extent are you willing to compromise what is most true and valuable for you? When you die, how important do you imagine it will be for you to feel that you have lived the life you most truly wished to live? How important that you feel you have fulfilled your potential?

Having been reminded of my mortality—the finite nature of being in this form—I can no longer imagine that there will always be a tomorrow. A greater sense of urgency has entered my approach to fulfilling my potential. Paradoxically, this includes a ruthless focus on being relaxed, at ease, and "in joy," letting go of ideas of fulfilling potential. More delicious paradox!

If a conversation bores me or a person's attitude creates an unpleasant feeling in me, then I am gone. If a party or book or film is not nourishing my soul, then I do not wait for the end before I end my involvement with it. We are each responsible for our moment-to-moment joy and well-being, and clearly no one else can take care of this for us. What I hope you will be able to see clearly is that your life circumstance and mine are not so different—I might die in a month or a few years or in a few decades ... I don't know. Statistically, having a brain tumor would mean there is an increased probability I will be dead in the next ten years; however, the fundamental truth of my life and yours is the same. So, what is important now?

I chose to get up at five o'clock this morning so I could give myself the treat of time to practice some qi gong and meditate before writing this chapter. I could have stayed in bed, or gone straight to breakfast after meditation, yet I find myself here in front of the computer, writing. Doing it rather than talking about it. I talked about writing a book for ten years, and whilst I did actually write here and there, I had no book to show for it. Now, as a result of asking myself this question more keenly and consistently, I have published my first book, my second is on the way. In addition, I contribute to creating companies and communities to facilitate human thriving. My answer to that big question is ever more one that I am satisfied with.

Perfectly Imperfect

An important point to note is that, for me, having fun and being in joy and in a relaxed state of healing is more important than anything else. I want to share as well that all the wonderful creativity and abundance that flows into my life now has happened despite periods when I allowed my answer to stem from greed, emotional reactivity, and other conditioned brain activity and tendencies of mind. The point I want to make is that the urgency and profound importance of the question needs to be balanced with a lightness of heart. Our efforts to be all that we can be need to be tempered with a recognition that, beyond this relative dance, we are perfect as we are. This is the nature of both personal and collective evolution—perfection is ever becoming more perfect. As Oscar Wilde noted, "Life is far too important to be taken seriously." So, please, let us be kind and gentle with ourselves. Let us enjoy both being and becoming.

Let us ask, "So, what is important now?"

Exercises

- *Imagine you have just discovered the world is going to be destroyed by a meteorite in six months' time. Alas, it is unavoidable, and the entire planet will be destroyed overnight. Write out what you will do with the next six months.*
- *Your fairy godmother is real and paying you a one-time visit. She will grant you everything you wish to be experiencing, creating, pursuing, exploring, and expressing; however, it's a one-shot deal, so don't hold back. Write out the life you should be*

*living—your ideal life that will bring you joy as
you describe it now. What sort of relationships
would you be enjoying? Which relationships
would be healed? Who would you forgive? What
type of work would you be doing? Where might
you travel to? What creative and self-expressive
pursuits would engage you?*

- *Looking at the first two exercises in this list, what
is it inside you that prevents you from living
the life of your dreams? Think carefully, and
don't settle for an excuse. Instead, seek to see
how holding certain beliefs about yourself and
the world—perhaps succumbing to fears and
doubts—has thus far created a distance between
your dreamed-of life and what you live. What
excites you about the prospect of changing?*
- *What can you do in the next twenty-four hours and
then on a daily basis for the next six weeks in
order to remove the obstructions you have created
and begin to live a more deeply fulfilling life?*

*Go confidently in the direction of
your dreams.
Live the life you've imagined.*

—Henry David Thoreau

Acknowledgments

This book being in your hands is thanks to many people including the editors Shanti Einolander, Jan Howarth, Zelda Turner, and Irene Pizzie, formatting and layout Lisa Simmonds, cover design Mia Yatiswara and Rowan Attenborough. These talented people are responsible for making the book so beautiful and much better ordered than I alone could manage. All errors are mine.

The funding of the final stages of production came via a crowdfund where 128 generous beings gave their backing. I express my gratitude to each one with special mention to Gregor Drugowitsch, Paul and Jeannie McGillivray, Lan Diep, Conrad Schroeder, Kate Friendship, Angela Orfield, Gordan Mandich, Val Czepulkowski, Sara Trevelyan, Jack Noble, Sinead Myerscough, Simon Milton and Robb Drury.

Those who gave feedback and impressions on the text, Ravi Gunaratnam, Nick Jankel especially, thank you.

To every author of every book I have read, including those in the small selection in the Further Reading section on the following pages, deep gratitude.

To those who have been so generous with their time in granting me interviews, Ken Wilber, Peter Russell, Amit Goswami, Martin Brofman, Anna Parkinson, Jun Po Denis Kelly Roshi, gratitude.

To my teachers, especially Jun Po Denis Kelly Roshi, Alan Seale, Mingtong Gu, Martin Brofman and Tracy Butler, great gratitude.

To my health and healing team, neurosurgeons, neurologists, anaesthetists, radiologists, oncologists, nurses, doctors, consultants, receptionists, naturopaths, energy healers, nutritionists, esoteric acupuncturists, herbalists, homeopaths, massage therapists, much gratitude.

To all my clients, students and workshop attendees, thank you for all you have taught me and for giving me the opportunity to be useful.

To business associates past and future, thank you.

To those angels who have graced this life, partners, lovers, girlfriends, eternal gratitude.

About the Author

Will Pye is a social entrepreneur, consultant, coach, speaker, and workshop leader. Having built companies within the charity fundraising sector, he currently works with individuals and groups globally facilitating the inner shifts which make the greatest difference.

Will is a practitioner of Zen, a student of *A Course in Miracles*, a yogi, a science geek, and was recently unwittingly initiated as a Sufi. He is a lover of Truth.

Will is the founder of The Love and Truth Project, a not-for-profit facilitating the emergence of a global community committed to allowing spiritual awakening to manifest through creative, environmental, and social justice projects. At its heart is a multi-faceted social experiment designed to create shifts in consciousness and culture utilizing the power of the transmission of higher states of consciousness.

He divides his time between Melbourne, Australia and Cambridge, England and regularly travels to North America and Europe offering meetings and workshops.

He can be reached at will@willpye.com

www.willpye.com

www.blessedwithabraintumor.com

www.loveandtruthproject.org

If this book has been useful please help spread the love and post a review on Amazon or share with your friends on social media. In gratitude.

Further Reading

Towards a More Scientific Worldview

Austin, James H. *Meditating Selflessly: Practical Neural Zen*. The MIT Press, 2013.

Bohm, David. *Wholeness and the Implicate Order*. Routledge, 2002.

Childre, Doc, and Howard Martin, with Donna Beech. *The HeartMath Solution: The Institute of HeartMath's Revolutionary Program for Engaging the Power of the Heart's Intelligence*. HarperOne, 2011.

Church, Dawson. *The Genie in Your Genes: Epigenetic Medicine and the New Biology of Intention*. Energy Psychology Press, 2009.

Doidge, Norman. *The Brain That Changes Itself: Stories of Personal Triumph from the Frontiers of Brain Science*. Penguin, 2008.

Goswami, Amit. *Self-Aware Universe: How Consciousness Creates the Material World*. Jeremy P. Tarcher, 1993.

Goswami, Amit. *God Is Not Dead: What Quantum Physics Tells Us about Our Origins and How We Should Live*. Hampton Roads Publishing Company, 2012.

Hanson, Rick. *Buddha's Brain: The Practical*

Neuroscience of Happiness, Love, and Wisdom. New Harbinger Publications, 2009.

Hood, Bruce. *The Self Illusion: Why There is No 'You' Inside Your Head*. Constable, 2012.

Lipton, Bruce. *The Biology of Belief: Unleashing the Power of Consciousness, Matter & Miracles*. Hay House, 2011.

McTaggart, Lynne. *The Field: The Quest for the Secret Force of the Universe*. Element, 2003.

McTaggart, Lynne. *The Bond: The Power of Connection*. Hay House, 2013.

Pert, Candace. *Molecules of Emotion: Why You Feel the Way You Feel*. Pocket Books, 1999.

Radin, Dean. *Entangled Minds*. Pocket Books, 2006.

Radin, Dean. *Conscious Universe: The Scientific Truth of Psychic Phenomena*. HarperOne, 2009.

Rosenblum, Bruce, and Fred Kuttner. *Quantum Enigma: Physics Encounters Consciousness*. Oxford University Press, 2011.

Talbot, Michael. *The Holographic Universe: The Revolutionary Theory of Reality*. Harper Perennial, 2011.

Creating Physical Health and Healing

Benson, Herbert. *The Relaxation Response*. Avon Books, 2000.

Brofman, Martin.* *Anything Can Be Healed*. Findhorn Press Ltd., 2003.

Chopra, Deepak. *Quantum Healing: Exploring the*

Frontiers of Mind/Body Medicine. Bantam, 1990.

Eden, Donna. *Energy Medicine: Balancing Your Body's Energies for Optimum Health, Joy and Vitality*. Piatkus, 2008.

Gawler, Ian.* *You Can Conquer Cancer*. Michelle Anderson Publishing, 2002.

Goswami, Amit. *The Quantum Doctor: A Quantum Physicist Explains the Healing Power of Integrative Medicine*. Hampton Roads Publishing, 2011.

Hamilton, David. *How Your Mind Can Heal Your Body*. Hay House, 2008.

Hay, Louise. *You Can Heal Your Life*. Hay House, 1984.

McTaggart, Lynne. *What Doctors Don't Tell You: The Truth about The Dangers of Modern Medicine*. Avon, 1999.

Ober, Clinton, Stephen T. Sinatra, and Martin Zucker. *Earthing: The Most Important Health Discovery Ever?* Basic Health Publications, 2010.

Parkinson, Anna.* *Change Your Mind, Heal Your Body: When Modern Medicine Has No Cure the Answer Lies Within. My True Story of Self-Healing*. Watkins Publishing, 2014.

Rankin, Lissa. *Mind Over Medicine: Scientific Proof That You Can Heal Yourself*. Hay House, 2013.

Servan-Schreiber, David. *Anticancer: A New Way of Life*. Michael Joseph, 2011.

Shealy, C. Norman. *Miracles Do Happen: A Physician's Experience with Alternative Medicine*. Element Books, 1995.

Siegel, Bernie. *Love, Medicine and Miracles*. Rider, 1999.

Simonton, O. Carl, Stephanie Matthews-Simonton, and
     James L. Creighton. *Getting Well Again: A Step-
     by-step, Self-help Guide to Overcoming Cancer for
     Patients and Their Families*. Bantam Books, 1986.
Turner, Kelly. *Radical Remission: Surviving Cancer
     Against All Odds*. HarperOne, 2014.

* Audio interviews with these authors are available at
     www.blessedwithabraintumor.com

Spirituality

Adyashanti. *Resurrecting Jesus: Embodying the Spirit of a
     Revolutionary Mystic*. Sounds True Inc., 2014.
Atkinson, William Walker, and the Three Initiates. *Kybalion:
     The Definitive Edition*. Jeremy P. Tarcher, 2011.
Beck, Charlotte J. *Everyday Zen*. HarperOne, 2007.
Blofeld, John (transl.). *The Zen Teaching of Huang Po:
     On the Transmission of Mind*. Grove Press/Atlantic
     Monthly Press, 2006.
Brown, Michael. *The Presence Process: A Journey into
     Present Moment Awareness*. Namaste Publishing
     Inc., 2010.
Caplan, Mariana. *Halfway Up the Mountain: The Error
     of Premature Claims to Enlightenment*. Hohm
     Press, 1999.
Caplan, Mariana. *Eyes Wide Open: Cultivating Discernment
     on the Spiritual Path*. Sounds True Inc., 2009.
Cleary, Thomas (transl.). *Shōbōgenzō: Zen Essays by
     Dogen*. University of Hawaii Press, 1992.

Ferrini, Paul. *Love Without Conditions (Reflections of the Christ Mind)*. Heartways Press, 1994.

Foundation for Inner Peace. *A Course in Miracles: Combined Volume*. Foundation for Inner Peace, 2008.

Frazier, Jan. *When Fear Falls Away: The Story of a Sudden Awakening*. Weiser Books, 2007.

Freke, Tim. *The Mystery Experience: A Revolutionary Approach to Spiritual Awakening*. Watkins Publishing Ltd., 2012.

Gross, Jonathan Paul.*The Great Doubt: Spirituality Beyond Dogma*. CreateSpace Independent Publishing Platform, 2011.

Hawley, Jack. *The Bhagavad Gita: A Walkthrough for Westerners*. New World Library, 2011.

Kapleau, Roshi P. *The Three Pillars of Zen: Teaching, Practice, and Enlightenment*. Anchor, 1989.

Kelly, Jun Po Denis, and Keith Martin-Smith. *The Heart of Zen: Enlightenment, Emotional Maturity, and What It Really Takes for Spiritual Liberation*. North Atlantic Books, 2014.

Katie, Byron, and Stephen Mitchell. *Loving What Is: Four Questions That Can Change Your Life*. Three Rivers Press, 2003.

Kautz, William H. *The Story of Jesus: An Intuitive Anthology*. Trafford Publishing, 2012.

Kornfield, Jack. *After the Ecstasy, the Laundry*. Bantam, 2001.

Kornfield, Jack. *A Path with Heart*. Rider, 2002.

Krishnamurti, Jiddu. *As One Is: To Free the Mind From*

All Conditioning. Hohm Press, 2007.

Maitland, Hokaku Jeffrey. *Mind, Body, Zen: Waking Up to Your Life*. North Atlantic Books, 2010.

Mitchell, Stephen (transl.). Lao Tsu, *Tao Te Ching*. Harper Collins, 1988.

McKenna, Jed. *Jed McKenna's Theory of Everything: The Enlightened Perspective*. Wisefool Press, 2013.

Nyland, A. *The Gospel of Thomas*. CreateSpace Independent Publishing Platform, 2011.

Packer, Toni. *The Work of This Moment*. Shambhala Publications Inc., 2007.

Roberts, Bernadette. *The Experience of No-Self: A Contemplative Journey*. State University of New York Press, 1993.

Sanchez, Nouk, and Tomas Vieira. *Take Me to Truth: Undoing the Ego*. John Hunt Publishing, 2007.

Thoreau, Henry David. *Walden (or Life in the Woods)*. Ticknor and Fields, 1854.

Wilber, Ken. *Integral Spirituality: A Startling New Role for Religion in the Modern and Postmodern World*. Shambhala Publications Inc., 2007.

Wiman, Christian. *My Bright Abyss: Meditation of a Modern Believer*. Farrar Straus Giroux, 2013.

Science and Spirituality Singing a Similar Song

Avery, Samuel. *Buddha and the Quantum: Hearing the Voice of Every Cell*. Sentient Publications, 2011.

Collins, Francis. *The Language of God: A Scientist Presents Evidence for Belief*. Pocket Books, 2007.

Dowd, Michael. *Thank God for Evolution: How the Marriage of Science and Religion Will Transform Your Life and Our World*. Plume, 2009.

McFarlane, Thomas J. (ed.) *Einstein and Buddha: The Parallel Sayings*. Ulysses Press, Seastone, 2002.

Polkinghorne, John. *Science and Religion in Quest of Truth*. SPCK Publishing, 2011.

Russell, Peter. *From Science to God: A Physicist's Journey into the Mystery of Consciousness*. New World Library, 2005.

Teilhard de Chardin, Pierre. *The Phenomenon of Man*. Harper and Brothers, 1959.

Wilber, Ken. *Quantum Questions: Mystical Writings of the World's Great Physicists*. Shambhala Publications Inc., 2001.

Psychology, Emotional Integration, and Shadow Work

Brown, Michael. *The Presence Process: A Journey into Present Moment Awareness*. Namaste Publishing Inc., 2010.

Ford, Debbie. *Dark Side of the Light Chasers: Reclaiming Your Power, Creativity, Brilliance, and Dreams*. Hodder Paperbacks, 2001.

Johnson, Robert A. *Owning Your Own Shadow: Understanding the Dark Side of the Psyche*.

HarperSanFrancisco, 1994.

Jung, Carl. (Aniela Jaffé, ed.; Clara Winston, transl.; Richard Winston, transl.) *Memories, Dreams, Reflections*. Vintage, 1989.

Lazaris. *Working With Your Shadow: An Imperative on the Spiritual Path*. NPN Publishing, Inc., 1995.

Ortner, Nick. *The Tapping Solution: A Revolutionary System for Stress-Free Living*. Hay House, 2014.

Riso, Don, and Russ Hudson. *The Wisdom of the Enneagram: The Complete Guide to Psychological and Spiritual Growth for the Nine Personality Types*. Bantam USA, 1999.

Rogers, Carl R. *On Becoming a Person: A Therapist's View of Psychotherapy*. Houghton Mifflin, 1995.

Siegel, Daniel J. *Mindsight: The New Science of Personal Transformation*. Bantam, 2010.

Wilber, Ken. *Integral Psychology: Consciousness, Spirit, Psychology, Therapy*. Shambhala Publications Inc., 2000.

Zweig, Connie, and Jeremiah Abrams (eds.) *Meeting the Shadow: The Hidden Power of the Dark Side of Human Nature*. Tarcher, 1991.

Death and Dying

Alexander, Eben. *Proof of Heaven: A Neurosurgeon's Journey into The Afterlife*. Piatkus, 2012.

Kübler-Ross, Elisabeth. *On Death and Dying*. Simon and Schuster, 2011.

Moody, Raymond A. *Life After Life*. Rider, 2001.

Moorjani, Anita. *Dying to Be Me: My Journey from Cancer, to Near Death, to True Healing.* Hay House, 2012.

van Lommel, Pim. *Consciousness Beyond Life: The Science of Near-Death Experience.* HarperOne, 2011.

Synchronicity

Chopra, Deepak. *Synchrodestiny: Harnessing the Infinite Power of Coincidence to Create Miracles.* Rider, 2005.

Combs, Allan, and Mark Holland. *Synchronicity: Through the Eyes of Science, Myth, and the Trickster.* Da Capo Press Inc., 2001.

Jaworski, Joseph. *Synchronicity: The Inner Path of Leadership.* Berrett-Koehler Publishers, 2011.

Jung, Carl. *Synchronicity: An Acausal Connecting Principle.* Routledge, 1985

Koestler, Arthur. *The Roots of Coincidence.* Random House, 1973.

Main, Roderick. *Revelations of Chance: Synchronicity as Spiritual Experience.* State University of New York, 2007.

Surprise, Kirby. *Synchronicity: The Art of Coincidence, Choice, and Unlocking Your Mind.* New Page Books, 2012.

Creating a New Reality/Birthing a New World

Dyer, Wayne W. *Manifest Your Destiny: The Nine Spiritual Principles for Getting Everything You Want*. William Morrow Paperbacks, 1998.

Eisenstein, Charles. *Sacred Economics: Money, Gift and Society in the Age of Transition*. Evolver Editions, 2011.

Eisenstein, Charles. *The More Beautiful World Our Hearts Know is Possible*. North Atlantic Books, 2013.

Hawken, Paul. *Blessed Unrest: How the Largest Social Movement in History is Restoring Grace, Justice, and Beauty to the World*. Penguin Books, 2008.

Hicks, Esther and Jerry. *Ask and It Is Given: Learning to Manifest Your Desires*. Hay House UK, 2010.

Johnson, Kurt, and David Robert Ord. *The Coming Interspiritual Age*. Namaste Publishing, 2013.

Seale, Alan. *Create a World That Works: Tools for Personal and Global Transformation*. Weiser Books, 2011.

Biographies

Frankl, Viktor E. *Man's Search for Meaning*. Rider & Co., 2008.

Gandhi, M. K. (Mahadev Desai, transl.) *An Autobiography: The Story of My Experiments with*

Truth. CreateSpace Independent Publishing Platform, 2011.

Isaacson, Walter. *Einstein: His Life and Universe*. Pocket Books, 2008.

Krakauer, Jon. *Into The Wild*. Pan, 2007.

Martin-Smith, Keith. *A Heart Blown Open: The Life and Practice of Zen Master Jun Po Denis Kelly Roshi*. Divine Arts, 2012.

Paramahansa Yogananda. *Autobiography of a Yogi*. Self-Realization Fellowship, 2006.

Schrödinger, Erwin. *What is Life?: With Mind and Matter and Autobiographical Sketches*. Cambridge University Press, 2012.

Thornton, Edward. *The Diary of a Mystic – A Rare Combination: Successful Business Man and Mystic*. George Allen & Unwin, 1967.

Bolte Taylor, Jill. *My Stroke of Insight: A Brain Scientist's Personal Journey*. Plume, 2009.

Poetry to Live By

Blake, William. *The Complete Poems*. Penguin Classics, 1977.

Hafiz. (Daniel Ladinsky, transl.) *The Gift – Poems by Hafiz the Great Sufi Master*. Penguin Compass, 1999.

Rumi, Jelaluddin. (Coleman Barks, transl.) *The Essential Rumi*. HarperOne, 2004.

DVD

Healing: Miracles, Mysteries and John of God. David
    Unterberg and Harald Wiesleitner, dirs., 2008.
The Living Matrix. Greg Becker, dir., 2009.
Sacred Science. Nicholas Polizzi, dir., 2011.
What the Bleep Do We Know?! William Arntz, Betsy
    Chasse, and Mark Vicente, dirs., 2004.

CPSIA information can be obtained at www.ICGtesting.com
Printed in the USA
BVOW08s1738260814

364231BV00005B/13/P